The Daily Tel

H
REPLACE

The Daily Telegraph

HIP
REPLACEMENT

THOMAS CRUMP

ROBINSON
London

Constable & Robinson Ltd
3 The Lanchesters
162 Fulham Palace Road
London W6 9ER
www.constablerobinson.com

First published in the UK by Robinson,
an imprint of Constable & Robinson Ltd, 2004

A copy of the British Library Cataloguing in Publication Data
is available from the British Library.

Publisher's Note: This book is not intended to be a substitute for medical
advice or treatment. Any person with a condition requiring medical
attention should consult a qualified medical practitioner
or suitable therapist.

ISBN 1-84119-664-9

Printed and bound in the EU

10 9 8 7 6 5 4 3 2 1

Contents

Acknowledgements

Many people have helped me both with my own total hip replacement (THR) and with writing this book. First come the two surgeons mentioned in the Introduction; Sarah Muirhead-Allwood in London and Piet de Bruyn in Tiel, who found in me a critical patient ready to ask any number of difficult questions. At a much later stage, James Scott FRCS invited me to visit him at the London offices of the *Journal of Bone and Joint Surgery* (of which he is one of the editors): I am extremely grateful for the way that he then, and later on, answered my most searching questions.

Professor Ian Learmonth FRCS, of the University of Bristol Department of Orthopaedic Surgery, provided most useful information about the choice of anaesthetics. An invitation to visit Richard Field FRCS, head of the Orthopaedic Research and Outcome Unit at St Helier's Hospital, Carshalton, led to invaluable information not only about developments at the cutting edge of THR, but also the post-operative outcome as experienced by patients. Last but not least, Richard Villar FRCS, Clinical Director of BUPA's Cambridge Hip and Knee Unit, invited me to be present in the operating theatre of the Cambridge Lea Hospital while he carried out a total hip replacement and then a revision knee replacement.

Leonard van Hogen, consultant anaesthetist at the Rivierland Ziekenhuis, was not only a mine of information when it came to the choice between different types of anaesthesia, but also a great comfort to me as I waited for the operation. For such support I am equally grateful to my own GP, Dr H.J.P.N. Land. Robert Royce of BUPA produced a wealth of information relating not only to insurance cover for THRs, but also to the way they were fitted into the operating programmes of hospitals, both NHS and private. Mike Tuke, Chief Executive of Finsbury Orthopaedics, invited me to his factory in Leatherhead, to observe the design and manufacture of prostheses, a field in which he is recognized as one of the leading figures.

Philip Batty of Paul Hartmann Ltd, a leading manufacturer of surgical supplies, told me in detail what was needed in the operating theatre for a THR. Jim Northcott, a very old friend, produced valuable material relating to the social and economic implications. Another old friend, Freda Dazeley MBE, told me how the Home Help Service cares for patients after discharge from hospital. Adrian Whitfield QC related THRs to possible legal actions for medical negligence. To all of these, and many others too numerous to mention, I am most grateful.

It may seem odd, but I received considerable help from Sweden, a country which I have only visited once, back in 1976, long before I had any hip problems. Sweden was already in the forefront of Charnley THRs, although the number of operations carried out by present-day standards was small. (In 1976 the number was less than 3,000; a quarter of a century later, in 2001, it was more than 12,000. The population of Sweden is about 15 per cent of that of the United Kingdom, so at this rate 80,000 THRs should be carried out, every year, in British hospitals; as I have already noted on page 110, the actual figure is almost certainly lower.)

Not only has Sweden an exceptionally strong THR record, but it also has the Swedish National Hip Arthroplasty Register, with its own website kept up to date by a team led by two professors of orthopaedic surgery from the University of Göteborg Medical School. As of writing, the Register analyses – in considerable detail – some 203,625 THRs, covering the years 1979–2001; since every orthopaedic department in Sweden contributes to the Register, there can be very few THRs not covered by it.

No other country has anything comparable to the Swedish Register. In the UK a number of hospitals have kept detailed records of THRs, and in others individual surgeons have done the same, but because the numbers of cases are inevitably much smaller, the information provided is less useful. The Swedish Register still defines the benchmarks for the long-term analysis of THRs; throughout this book I have used it in this spirit, at the same time taking into account the differences – in surgical practice, demography, social services, health care provision and so on – between Sweden and the UK. (I have been assured that the community of British orthopaedic surgeons shares my admiration for what their Swedish colleagues have achieved.)

Although I could hardly have written this book without my own experience as a patient, much of my material is the result of research carried out in the libraries of the Charing Cross Hospital in London and the Academic Medical Centre in Amsterdam. Both are world-class medical schools and I am most grateful to their library staff for the help given to me.

Foreword

Those contemplating the need for a total hip replacement (THR) will be reassured to know that the operation is straightforward, it works and it lasts. The principle behind the procedure is obvious enough. The underlying problem in hip arthritis is the erosion with time of the smooth cartilage that covers the surface of the femur and the cup into which it fits – thus exposing the bone underneath. So, rather than two glistening surfaces rolling smoothly over each other, bone grinds on bone. The result is a constant nagging pain which perplexingly is often worse at night. Further, the pain and stiffness of the hips alters the biomechanics of the whole skeleton causing additional symptoms in the lower back and down towards the knees.

Back in the late 1960s a British orthopaedic surgeon of genius, John Charnley, devised an operation in which he cut away the arthritic hip and replaced it with an artificial ball and socket that he had designed to replicate the joints' two vital and contradictory attributes – of both maintaining the weight of the body while at the same time ensuring full mobility. His total hip replacement proved to be one of the most reliably successful operations ever conceived, so successful indeed that 70,000 people in Britain this year alone will benefit from it.

This very success, however, as Thomas Crump points out, produces several difficulties of its own to which his book draws attention and seeks to resolve. First, there is, not surprisingly, an enormous demand for the operation precisely because it works so well – but the number of orthopaedic surgeons is necessarily limited. Thus, as many will find, they must wait eighteen months or more before their number comes up, and that can be very onerous. The lengthy waiting list in turn requires the surgeons to speed patients through the system so there is not, as there was in the past, the time or opportunity for patients to stay long enough in hospital for them to regain full mobility. Then again while the Total Hip Replacement is remarkably safe, it will inevitably cause complications in a minority that it is always useful to anticipate.

Thomas Crump's book, drawing on his own experience of the operation, addresses all these questions in turn in the hope of maximizing the chances that, as he found, it is as trouble-free as possible. He draws attention to several dodges for negotiating the waiting list including the option of 'going private' whose merits and disadvantages he judiciously compares. Then the rapid hospital turn around necessarily shifts the responsibility to rehabilitation back on to the patient so appropriately he devotes several pages to the sort of exercises that are necessary to strengthen muscular power and joint mobility.

Next, while the risk of THP may be gratifyingly small this does not mean that the complications that can occur – notably infection and loosening of ther prosthesis – may not be very serious. Thomas Crump's own experience, like that of 95 per cent of patients, proved to be devoid of these complications – but, by the same token, it is only sensible to know what you are letting yourself in for and thus be prepared for any hazards that may intervene.

Hip Replacement is set apart from most books on health matters as it is written by a distinguished historian of science whose personal experience of the operation is complemented by a thorough research into his subject. It can be commended not just as a comprehensive patient oriented introduction to the subject, but also as 'a good read'.

James Le Fanu

Introduction

'Total hip and total knee replacement have probably improved the quality and quantity of life in the Western world, more than any other single medical technology in the history of mankind.'

Dane Miller, Orthopaedic surgeon

This is a book about total hip replacement (THR), a major surgical operation carried out every year in the United Kingdom on some 70,000 patients. Given the average NHS waiting time, the number of people waiting for such an operation may be even greater. In the world as a whole the number of operations may be more than a million per annum. The operation relieves arthritis of the hip by replacing the joint affected with a prosthesis, a manufactured implant made of specially developed durable inorganic materials.

THR, as a viable operation, is hardly thirty years old. Sixty years ago I started at a new school, where my

50-year-old form-master, Bill Cheesman, was crippled by arthritis of the hip. He was unlucky to suffer so young, but as a young man he had been a star rugby player, so he belonged to a high-risk category. I can still remember how he would lumber into the classroom, helped by a stick, and with difficulty take the two steps up to the podium where he had his desk.

All this was in 1943, and although Bill Cheesman lived until 1969, it is unlikely that anything was ever done to improve his condition. Today, even with NHS waiting lists, a THR operation would have given him almost 100 per cent relief from the considerable pain and discomfort he suffered and the last third of his life would have been transformed.

In this book I want to help all of you who suffer from arthritis of the hips come to terms with THR, which in the long run is the only effective means of relieving the pain, discomfort and lack of mobility. (I use 'arthritis' where the medical profession would prefer the more general term 'arthrosis'. In medicine, arthritis means *inflammation* of a joint, which in most THR cases is absent.)

I had the operation in November 2001, by which time I had been suffering from arthritis of the hip for more than two years. Following the operation I experienced the improved quality of life claimed for it by Dr Miller, who is quoted at the head of this chapter.

This book confirms how THR relates to many different aspects of life, of which the patient's medical history is only part. And even when it comes to the medical side, the surgeon is far from being the only person involved. In researching this book I have talked with any number of orthopaedic surgeons, and time and again I was referred elsewhere. At the same time the surgeons, surprisingly often, contradicted each other.

'You must ask the anaesthetist/physiotherapist/your insurance company . . . that question' was all too often the answer I was given by a surgeon. It is astonishing how compartmentalized the medical world is, which is part of the problem when it is a question of such radical treatment as a THR. All too often, too many people are involved, and there are numerous breakdowns in communication.

Any major operation is the work of quite a large team, which in all too many orthopaedic departments has to be reconstituted for every single operation. From what I have seen, the best-case scenario is to be found where the team is kept together for a whole series of total hip replacements, performed in the course of one or two days (together, perhaps, with a number of knee replacements). At the same time, it helps if the hospital has separate wards for trauma and elective surgery patients (to which class those awaiting a THR belong). Otherwise, trauma patients (often first treated by Accident and Emergency) are only too likely to crowd out those awaiting elective surgery. There is also some risk of cross-infection.

John Charnley, whose story is told in Chapter 3, and who may prove to be the all-time top-scorer, thought nothing of carrying out nine THRs in a single day. There is no doubt that he, and no one else, called the shots at his hospital in Wrightington.

Because of the long waiting lists, I, like many others, opted for private treatment and I was booked for surgery by Sarah Muirhead-Allwood FRCS on 14 November 2001. A pre-operative consultation three weeks before the due date taught me an immense amount about THR. I was particularly impressed by the mechanical precision with which the operation was planned by a leading specialist, internationally known for her skill in hip surgery. It was not to be, however. I live in Holland, and in spite of their legal obligations as stated by the European Court (see Chapter 11) my Dutch insurance company did everything to prevent an operation in England. At the last moment they found Piet de Bruyn (who had trained in England and had attended the odd Wrightington seminar given by John Charnley at the end of the 1970s), and I was booked for an operation by him in the Rivierland Ziekenhuis at the end of November. (This hospital, in the small Dutch town of Tiel, would also welcome British NHS patients for THR.)

The question is this: how much difference does it make to be operated on in Holland (or any other EU country) rather than in the United Kingdom? The answer is, not much. Dutch and British surgeons may prefer different approaches to the actual hip-joint, but both would accept that this was mainly a question of what one was used to. In special cases each would have little difficulty in adopting an alternative approach. To the anaesthetized patient it does not make any difference either way. Nor does it make any difference to the process of recovery.

The main difference is the continental preference for local rather than general anaesthesia. This case is argued in Chapter 7, but the results are largely inconclusive. (Some specialists claim that the British practice makes it almost certain that the patient will require a blood transfusion – which the Dutch often avoid. Others doubt whether the preference for general anaesthesia is a key factor here).

The position is far from being cut and dried: in both the Netherlands and the United Kingdom both types of anaesthesia are used where appropriate, and every orthopaedic department will have its own criteria for the decision made in any particular case.

> Orthopaedic surgeons and anaesthetists belong to an international community. To give one example, surgeons from many different countries (almost certainly including Holland) will have attended the conference on hip surgery held in Edinburgh in September 2002. What they learnt from each other could certainly be carried out in practice in their own countries. This is the way that John Charnley's THR became standard surgical practice throughout the world. That is what such meetings are for, and the Edinburgh conference was just one of many devoted to hip surgery held in different parts of the world.

My THR was a textbook case, in spite of possible complications arising from Perthes' disease, a condition of the upper femur (described briefly in Chapter 1) from which I had suffered as a child in the 1930s. Like some 95 per cent of patients everywhere I suffered none of the possible complications described in Chapter 7. I was discharged within a week, walking without crutches within two weeks and driving the car within three. I was a new man.

Unfortunately, for some of you who are reading this book – while waiting for a THR – this will be too good to be true. Your recovery may not be so rapid or straightforward, the operation is not all plain sailing. The best I can do is point out the hazards and tell you how they are dealt with. I share the optimism expressed in the quotation at the head of this chapter – at the same time asking those of you whose THR proves to be more problematic not to hold it against me.

Every patient is a separate case and every surgeon has his own approach to the operation. The two together are not always the right combination, and this may be a reason for things going wrong without any obvious mistakes being made. Both patients and surgeons are human, though one might not think so from some of the published material on THR – which make it sound like a production-line operation (almost certainly how it is treated in the computerized accounting of the NHS).

Nevertheless procedures do tend to be standardized, for although prostheses come in a number of different sizes, and are made of different materials, the operation described in Chapter 7 is essentially the only way of implanting them.

In writing this book I have done my best to look at THR, and the condition it is designed to cure, from every angle that could be relevant to you as a patient.

In Chapter 1, I explain how you as a patient can tell whether you are suffering from arthritis of the hip, and then go on to describe what this involves for your own body.

Chapter 2 explores possible means of relieving your suffering, without resorting to surgery. In this chapter I also note (with some scepticism) how alternative medicine may even cure the arthritis in your hip without surgery.

At first you may find Chapter 3 something of a digression. Why do you need to know about one man, the orthopaedic surgeon John Charnley? After all you can switch on an electric light bulb without knowing anything about Thomas Edison, who invented it in the late nineteenth century. On the other hand, the ghost of Charnley still hovers over every THR. He would be just over ninety years old if he were still alive today. Your own surgeon may even have been trained by him – mine was. Quite simply, John Charnley solved almost all the key problems. If you read about the way he did so, after years of trial and disappointment, you will understand much better your own operation, and the results you can expect from it.

In Chapter 4, I deal with what is an almost obsessive concern of many, if not most, THR patients. Once you are on track for a THR you will find yourself asking any number of questions beginning with 'when', or 'how long before . . .' In this chapter I do my best to answer them.

Chapter 5 you may find disconcerting, but its theme of 'risk' cannot be avoided. Even though THR is a remarkably successful operation, it is not always straightforward. If you are honest with yourself, you will want to know, beforehand, about the possible hazards.

After coming to terms with the time and risk factors, you will be concerned with what you must do as you wait for the operation. This is dealt with in Chapter 6, which focuses largely on preparations to be made for your return home after discharge from hospital.

Chapter 7 is the key to the whole book, because it describes the operation itself. Although the details are more the concern of the surgeon than of you, the patient, you may well be interested to know what is being done to you. This is all the more important given alternative procedures relating to such matters as the choice between local and general anaesthesia, or between cemented and uncemented implants. You may also have a say in the choice of prosthesis, including the possibility of the relatively new Birmingham Hip Resurfacing.

Chapter 8 tells you what you can expect as you recover from the operation, first in hospital and then at home. Every stage in the process is dealt with, including possible setbacks.

Chapter 9 is mainly concerned with the supporting services, often provided by your local council, that you can call on in the weeks and months following your THR. This chapter will particularly interest those of you who live alone, without being able to call on family, friends or neighbours for help in such everyday tasks as shopping.

A THR belongs to the domain of 'elective surgery' – because the operation is essentially non-urgent, it is only too easy to put the patient on hold. You may already have discovered the horrible truth about NHS waiting lists, whatever the government has promised to do about reducing them. Private treatment, the subject of Chapter 10, could well put an end to your sorrows, but it comes at a price, not only in terms of money but of the course of treatment. In extreme cases (such as are dealt with in Chapter 5) you may still land up in a NHS hospital.

Chapter 11 takes you a step further and tells you about treatment abroad (which may even be arranged through the NHS). The position here is uncertain, because your legal rights as a THR patient still await the outcome of litigation before the European Court.

From Chapter 12 you will learn what the future may have in store for you as a patient suffering from arthritis of the hip. In the short term the answer is not very much, but who knows what alternatives to conventional THR will be available in the more distant future?

Finally, I could not have written this book without experiencing, as a THR patient, many of the different problems that I discuss. Some of these are general, others relate to my own circumstances. It is appropriate, then, to say a word about my own THR in relation to my family, who had to look after me when, as a patient, I was in varying degrees incapacitated. Every day during my week in hospital I enjoyed visits from my wife Carolien, and my son Maarten and his wife Annet. When they had gone, I enjoyed long telephone calls with my daughter, Laurien, in England.

One of the sadder aspects of writing about THR is the need to accept that, for a variety of reasons, all too many of you as patients will not enjoy the same level of care and support from family and friends. I had you especially in mind when writing this book.

1
Suffering from Arthritis

It's All in our Joints

When something goes wrong and you find yourself less
mobile than you used to be, it is easy to be told 'it's in your
joints'. This is more than likely to be true, but it is small
consolation when you are suffering the agonies of arthritis,
the most common medical condition that causes pain in the
joints. The condition is particularly acute when it affects the
joints in our hips or knees, which must support the burden
of our walking, almost uniquely among animal species, on
two feet. Now, for little more than a generation, radical
surgery has been able to put an end to this form of arthritis.
This defines the subject matter of my book.

Moving Around

In common with all advanced living organisms, the basic
framework of our bodies consists of bones and muscles.

Bones form the skeleton and muscles produce movement of the body and maintain its position against the force of gravity. These together comprise the muscular-skeletal system, which in medical practice is largely the province of orthopaedics.

Significantly, *dōbutsu*, the Japanese word for 'animal', means a 'being that moves', in contrast to other forms of life, such as plants.

My focus in this book is on the movement of the thigh in relation to the hip, and the pathological conditions that this, in the long term of our human life span, can give rise to.

Movement is only possible because the skeleton is articulated, with adjacent bones, such as the femur and the pelvis, in contact at joints, but able to move independently of each other. The phenomenon is essentially mechanical. Our bones are massive and extremely durable. Although, as part of the human body, our skeleton is subject to continuous biological processes, it can be taken to be immutable – that is, the bones that comprise it do not change significantly from day to day. The position is different with growing children, who have their own orthopaedic problems, some of which, such as Perthes' disease (described on pages 22–3), may later cause arthritis of the hip. The condition itself hardly occurs in children or young adults.

Constant bodily movement means that the contact surfaces at the joints between our bones are continuously changing in relation to each other. Any such relative movement is resisted by friction. The result in our own bodies is that some of the energy required for movement (and transmitted to the skeletal system by muscles) is lost at the joints, to be converted into some other, unwanted, form of energy, such as heat. The discovery of such conversion, which goes back to the end of the eighteenth century, was a major breakthrough in the history of science. The medical implications only became clear in the twentieth century – largely as a result of the work of John Charnley.

Engineers designing mechanical systems are endlessly preoccupied with the problem of friction: the lubrication systems of the modern car are indispensable to its operation, and the same goes for almost any other mechanism with moving parts. Without lubrication two things would happen: excessive heat would be generated, and the contact surfaces would wear away, leaving debris in such forms as fine particles of metallic dust to clog up the mechanical system. At the same time the components degenerate, with inevitable loss of function.

Our Joints

How, then, does the mechanical system of the human skeleton deal with this problem at the points of articulation, known to all of us simply as 'joints'? To begin with, there must be a sufficiently good fit between the contact surfaces: the hip-joint, the crown of the femur, and the acetabulum, the corresponding part of the pelvis, constitute a ball and socket joint. In engineering the contact surfaces, ideally, are perfectly spherical, a result that precision machining comes close to attaining. The human body is less perfect, with the result that in any position of the thigh in relation to the hip, the actual contact area is relatively small.

It is critical, then, that the friction between the two surfaces, at their contact point, should be reduced to an absolute minimum. Here the Darwinian evolution of the human anatomy has achieved results better than anything reached by even the best contemporary engineering. This result is inherent in the mechanical characteristics of the contact surfaces at a joint. There our bones are covered with a protective layer of articular cartilage, which produces a shiny glasslike appearance (such as can be seen at the end of the bone in a chicken drum-stick). The layer of cartilage has also sufficient elasticity to ensure something better than a single point of contact at the joint. The synovium – that is the sac enclosing the joint – also contains a sort of grease (the synovial fluid) that helps smooth articulation. The friction between the two contact surfaces is then at such a low level that most of us do not even notice any unwanted conversion of energy when we move our limbs.

Unfortunately such good fortune does not always last a life time, particularly now when we live much longer than ever before. Arthritis is the most common cause of this misfortune.

The word arthritis means no more than inflammation of a joint, derived from the Greek word *arthron*. As noted in the Introduction, the term is not quite accurate, since in most cases inflammation is not part of the pathology: this is why doctors prefer the general term arthrosis.

Although in principle arthritis can afflict almost any joint, it is most likely to hit the joints subject to the greatest stress in everyday life. For our own two-legged species, this means the hip and the knee, which together are constantly called on to support the whole weight of our bodies. It is therefore important to understand the ways in which the hip can move, and the loading to which, as the largest joint in our bodies, it is subjected in every life.

The Movement of our Legs

The main back and forward movement of our leg, in relation to the body, is in the so-called *sagittal* plane: this is what an observer sees when looking from the side at someone walking.

The word actually derives from *sagitta*, Latin for 'arrow', whose trajectory is in this plane in relation to the archer.

A person walking straight forward moves in the sagittal plane, and in walking, the angle between the legs will be about 70 degrees at its maximum. This is by no means the maximum flexion possible, which with a healthy joint should be around 120 degrees.

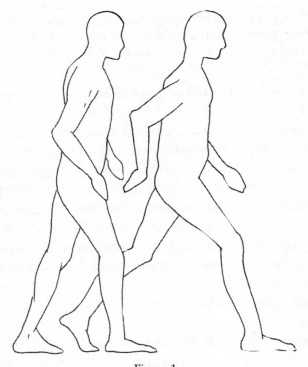

Figure 1

The main back and forward movement of the leg, in relation to the body, is in the sagittal plane, as shown in Figure 2 on page 18. This figure shows what an observer sees, when looking from the side, at a THR patient, before and after the operation.

Our legs can also move sideways in the *frontal* plane: moving inwards is called *adduction*, outwards, *abduction*. At the same time they can rotate in the transverse plane: *internal* rotation points the foot inwards, *external* rotation points it outwards. All four of these movements also occur in normal walking but only up to an angle of about 5 degrees; because this is but a fraction of the movement in the sagittal plane, we hardly notice it.

The action of muscles produces the movement in each of the three planes. This explains why the whole hip-joint is embedded in muscles, each with its own function. For example, flexion and internal rotation are controlled by muscles at the front of the hip, and extension and abduction by the three gluteal muscles which make up the buttocks. A major problem which a surgeon faces is to find the optimal approach, through the gluteal muscles, to the joint itself. Both arthritis of the hip and the surgery (THR) designed to relieve it can lead to the muscles becoming shorter: this is known as contracture. The most common form is flexion contracture, when bending the hip becomes difficult, and straightening it even more so.

As to the maximum freedom of movement, that in the frontal and transverse planes, although less than in the sagittal plane, is still considerable: Figure 2 shows the amount of freedom required for seven different types of everyday activity. With arthritis this freedom is considerably reduced, and you will find that these activities become progressively more difficult, to the point that some activities, such as tying shoelaces, become all but impossible. This will be noted also by the orthopaedic surgeon during your first consultation.

There is a wide range of loading conditions, each imposing its own stresses on the hip-joint. These range from 'lightly loaded high-speed motions such as in the swing phase of walking and running', through 'impact loads of short duration and large magnitude such as jumping', to 'fixed steady loads such as during prolonged standing'.

In terms of the standard gravitational pull, known

Activity	Plane of Motion	Recorded value (degrees)
Tying shoe with foot on floor	Sagittal Frontal Transverse	124 19 15
Tying shoe with foot crossed over opposite thigh	Sagittal Frontal Transverse	110 23 33
Sitting down on chair and rising from sitting	Sagittal Frontal Transverse	104 20 17
Stooping to pick up object from floor	Sagittal Frontal Transverse	117 21 18
Squatting	Sagittal Frontal Transverse	122 28 26
Going up stairs	Sagittal Frontal Transverse	67 16 18
Coming down statirs	Sagittal	36

Figure 2 *shows the amount of freedom required for seven different types of everyday activity according to the three planes in the human body.*

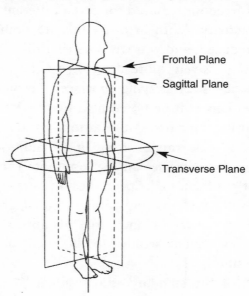

simply as G, these loading conditions require our hip-joints to withstand forces of up to 7G, and they are surprisingly often required to do so. They are therefore quite remarkably robust, so much so that most of us, even in these days of an ageing population, will never suffer from arthritis of the hip or knee. As a reader of this book, you probably belong to the considerable minority who do suffer.

The Origins of Hip Arthritis

The first question you may then want to ask is, quite simply, what went wrong? There is no single answer. Some of you (more women than men) will have joints where the protecting layer of cartilage has failed to stand up to the stresses of daily life. This is more likely to happen where the contact area between the two bones at the joint is relatively small. In some cases this will be the result of lifestyle earlier in life – in America high-school football players are a high-risk category, and in others specific conditions such as congenital acetabular dysplasia or Perthes' disease may be responsible. In most cases, however, there is no obvious explanation.

Failure is most likely to occur with old age, at a time of life when the biological processes that continuously restore damaged tissue slow down. Those of you who are over seventy-five years old should know that in this age group nearly 100 out of every 1,000 men suffer from arthritis and more than 200 out of every 1,000 women. Obesity is also likely to increase the risk of arthritis of the hip and is certainly a factor influencing the course of treatment.

When this stage has been reached, the cartilage will have worn away to the point that the bones comprising your affected hip-joint will be in direct contact. Cartilage will no longer ensure the low friction surface required for normal use of the limbs affected, so you will suffer from progressive loss of function and mobility. At the same time, you will experience an increasing level of pain, which with an arthritic hip can take various forms. Typically you will feel the pain at the groin on the side of the affected hip, and as radiated pain it may extend down the inside of the leg, even beyond the knee, or around the side of the thigh to the buttocks.

The pathology of arthritis – particularly as loss of freedom of movement – is likely to be present for some time before you feel any pain, and it is quite possible that normal bodily processes keep the condition under control in such a way that you are not even conscious of it. A mass X-ray programme would no doubt reveal many such cases, but the trouble and expense would hardly be justified, since with arthritis treatment is focused on the symptoms rather than prevention.

When symptoms do begin to appear, pain may be intermittent and not particularly severe, so that for weeks or even months you may live with the condition and hold back from consulting a doctor. Walking, particularly going up stairs, will become difficult, and the same applies to getting up from a chair, out of bed or into a car. There is no overall rate of deterioration:

your condition could become acute within weeks, but equally you could live in reasonable comfort for some years without treatment. In the process, your condition may well stabilize for quite long periods, followed by rapid deterioration.

Although arthrosis is primarily a condition suffered by the elderly, it does register, at a low level, in the statistics for the forty-five to sixty-five year age group. The figures per 1,000 people are 26 for men and 40 for women. The lifestyle of patients when young is much more likely to explain the early onset of arthrosis. Contact sports increase the risk of it occurring at a young age. The risk is high with other occupations, such as ballet dancing, which put excessive demands on the hip. Those working in agriculture are also more likely to suffer at a relatively young age. For such patients, a special operation, Birmingham Hip Resurfacing – so amed because it was developed by surgeons working in Birmingham – has been developed. (See page 107).

Surgical Treatment

Until some thirty years ago, if you suffered from arthritis of the hip you would just have had to live with it, sometimes for decades. The principle of 'grin and bear it' would have been little consolation, although painkillers, particularly those available only as prescription drugs, became steadily more effective. Then, in the course of the twenty years after 1950, effective surgery became possible. This was largely the achievement of one man, John Charnley, whose life's work is described in Chapter 3.

The treatment was radical. Both sides of the affected

hip-joint were removed, to be replaced by a prosthesis. This is why the operation (described in detail in Chapter 5) is popularly known as 'total hip replacement', THR for short.

The general condition, substantially alleviated by THR, is primary osteoarthritis. The word 'primary' means that it appears without any specific cause in the medical history of the patient. The prefix 'osteo' comes from the Greek *osteon*, which means simply 'bone', while *arthron* means 'joint', but only between bones.

Secondary osteoarthritis is often the result of a fracture, and in such cases the risk of it occurring later in life commonly provides a reason for immediate surgery rather than some form of conservative treatment. With a hip fracture this may provide the occasion for a THR, but even if it does not, a THR, as a result of secondary osteoarthritis, may still be necessary later in life.

The body of the 4,000-year-old Tyrolean ice-man, recently discovered in a remarkable state of preservation almost on the border between Austria and Italy, shows clear signs of secondary osteoarthritis – though not in the hip. With only prehistoric medicine to help him he must have suffered considerable pain.

Special Cases Indicating a THR

A number of specific and often uncommon bone conditions indicate that a THR, to cure osteoarthritis, will eventually become necessary. One of these is Perthes' disease, which afflicts the head of the femur. This is a rare condition, occurring in children between the ages of three and eight. Boys, particularly those who are short for their age, suffer more than girls.

The Perthes, symptoms are two fold: first, the leg afflicted is shorter than the other leg; second, there may be acute localized pain, either in the hip or the groin. The cause is a loss of circulation of blood to the head of the femur, during the period – generally something over a year – when the condition evolves. This means that the head of the femur becomes soft beneath the layer of cartilage, and so, with normal growth, the weight constantly placed upon it causes partial collapse. The degenerative process stops as a result of spontaneous remission. In other words, the condition – although various treatments can now relieve it – cures itself, but it will leave a legacy in the form of a non-spherical crown to the femur. The result will be a poor fit into the acetabulum, and a joint prone to arthritis.

Little is known about Perthes' disease and in many cases – particularly when onset occurs before the child's fourth birthday – no active treatment is necessary, and the boy or girl may well go through life without any pain or discomfort. In any case, nothing will restore the length lost to the shorter leg, or correct the deformation of the femur, both of which greatly increase the probability of osteoarthritis of the hip occurring later in life. The shorter leg can be helped by heightening the heel of shoes and other footwear, which may well delay the onset of arthritis, but nothing can be done about the deformation of the femur (which, of course, will disappear if and when a prosthesis is fitted as part of a THR).

Rheumatoid arthritis can also affect the hip-joint, and indicate a THR as the best treatment. Pathologically, there is a clear distinction between the two conditions. Rheumatoid arthritis, which affects more than 350,000 people in the UK, is an autoimmune disease afflicting the synovial lining of joints, and surgery is generally the last resort in treatment. At the same time the hip is seldom the primary site of the condition, so that of all the THRs carried out, very few relate directly to rheumatoid arthritis. A new drug, rituximab, also offers the prospect of effective treatment, so that THRs for rheumatoid arthritis patients are likely to become considerably less frequent.

Fractures around the hip-joint are often best treated with THR, particularly among elderly people. When – as often occurs – the femoral neck is fractured, the result is to interfere with the blood supply to the femoral crown. This leads not to osteoarthritis but to a condition known as avascular necrosis. The symptoms, in terms of pain, lack of function and mobility, are much the same, as is the relief provided by THR. With certain conditions affecting the structure of the bone, such as Paget's disease, minute stress fractures occur – a THR may then be the best means of preventing a complete fracture.

Summary

At the end of the day, although your own THR may have followed from one of the special cases described above, the chances are that you will be one of the great majority of patients for whom no specific cause of their arthritis can be found. Do not let this get you down. You are in good company and the relief following from a THR is the same. I speak from experience. I was a Perthes' disease patient, but this was only discovered when my first consultation with an orthopaedic surgeon made it clear that I should have a THR. This made no difference to the course of treatment, so that I became just one of the tens of thousands whose lives are transformed – as I hope yours will be – by having the operation.

2
Alternatives to Total Hip Replacement

Mainline medical care

Apart from THR surgery, no treatment for arthritis of the hip is completely effective. Nonetheless, such surgery is elective – that is, the final choice rests with you, the patient – and in certain cases it is simply too risky. In any case, with long waiting times for surgery, you are certainly right to be interested in any treatment that alleviates the condition, or is claimed to do so. At the same time you might be lucky in finding a local patient support group. The best starting point here is Arthritis Care, a national organization, based on London, but with eight regional offices. Its website address is www.arthritis.org.uk.

To begin with, the patient can take a number of steps to make life more tolerable without any medical supervision.

The first is to control one's weight. Here the Body Mass Index (BMI) is useful, although it does require patients to be conversant with the metric system of weights and measures. It also helps to have a pocket calculator.

To calculate your BMI, divide your weight in kilograms by the square of your height in metres. In my own case this means dividing 74 by the square of 1.70, so that 74 divided by 2.89 gives an index of 25.6. This is just inside the 25–30 range, which indicates overweight, but not to a degree that is cause for concern. If, however, my weight were 7 kilograms greater, and my height 6 centimetres less, then the index would be 30.5, and I would be classed as obese. I would then be well advised to reduce my weight in order to relieve the pain of arthritis. This would also have the advantage of making future surgery somewhat simpler, and reducing the risks accompanying it, to say nothing of the improvement in general health.

Force of circumstance, if nothing else, is likely to make you, as an arthritis sufferer, change your pattern of activity. This will affect sport and recreation, travel and your life at home. Tennis and ten-mile walks will be out, public transport will become problematic, and you will find chores at ground level – particularly in the garden – painful. Even standing for a few minutes will cause distress, which is frustrating when it comes to activities such as cooking. Carrying heavy objects will be difficult. As time goes by, you will adapt, walk with a stick and even carry a small folding stool. (Medical suppliers stock special lightweight models, but these are rather expensive.) When travelling, suitcases on wheels are indispensable and a walking stick is surprisingly effective in encouraging passengers to offer you their seats in public transport.

What is more, you will come to recognize your limitations, but these can vary considerably from one person to another. In the course of time, the limitations are likely to become more severe, with increasing levels of pain. This is the main reason why short waiting lists for THRs are so important, particularly if loss of function and mobility make it difficult for you to look after yourself.

The question is whether anything can be done to enhance function and mobility, or at least slow down the rate of deterioration. Here a positive attitude certainly helps. You should think more of what is still possible in normal life, and less of what has been lost. Swimming, for example, encourages many people at this stage, although stiff arthritic limbs are still a hindrance.

An American therapist, Lynda Huey, has even developed what she calls 'waterpower', as a fitness programme designed to avoid more radical treatment entirely. For its application to arthritis of the hip, she has joined up with Robert Klapper, an orthopaedic surgeon, to write a book. If you are interested in trying out waterpower, you should read *Heal Your Hips: How to Prevent Hip Surgery – and What to Do If You Need It.*

Another possibility is physiotherapy. This can take so many different forms that it is difficult to deal with them all. Massage and different sorts of manipulation may provide you with relief, and your physiotherapist may well be able to recommend helpful exercises still within your capacity. Although none of this will cure your condition, anything that can make your life more tolerable is worth trying. Here the experience of patients (and also the attitude of doctors) varies widely.

Medication

Medicines can substantially relieve the pain caused by arthritis. The most commonly used are NSAIDs, which is short for nonsteroidal anti-inflammatory drugs. These include such well-known drugs as aspirin, but for relieving the pain of arthritis ibuprofen is commonly prescribed, although it is sold with the trade names Brufen and Junifen. An alternative, Diclofenac, may be even more effective.

Effective drugs are mostly enzyme inhibitors, targeting one particular enzyme, which comes in two forms: COX-1 and COX-2. (Enzymes, of which there are many different types, are proteins active in the body which speed up the rate of biochemical reactions, without themselves being used up in the process.) It is the COX-2 reaction that causes the sensation of pain in arthritis of the hip. If, therefore, it can be inhibited, you will suffer less pain. The problem is that a drug such as ibuprofen also inhibits the COX-1 reactions, which are important in protecting the stomach lining from the action of digestive acids. This, then, limits the dosage level that can be safely prescribed, so that two tablets (7.5mg per tablet) per day are the maximum. There are, however, new drugs such as the American celecoxib (sold as Celebrex), which, by specifically targeting the COX-2 enzymes, are more effective as painkillers. Even so, recent research has caused doubts about their long-term effectiveness. They may also substantially increase the risk of a heart attack. Appropriate NSAIDs will probably make your life as an arthritis sufferer more bearable, but they will not stop the progressive loss of function and mobility, nor cure the condition that causes it.

Somewhat paradoxically, steroids, as well as NSAIDs, can be effective in counteracting inflammation, and thereby reducing pain. Cortisone, one of the naturally occurring hormones synthesized by the adrenal cortex (which is part of a gland just above the kidney), belongs to this group and so should be effective in cases of arthritis. Its side-effects, however, make it much less safe to prescribe than standard NSAIDs, so its use is much more restricted.

A much more radical treatment is the injection into the hip-joint of an appropriate steroid (hydrocortisone acetate or the long-acting triamcinolone) combined with a local anaesthetic. Although the results are sometimes miraculous, they are not very long-lasting and once again, because undesirable side-effects discourage continuing the injections indefinitely, they will not provide a long-term solution to your problem.

Arthroscopy and other Surgery

If you are under the age of 55 and retain a reasonable range of movement within the hip, a type of keyhole surgery known as arthroscopy offers you an alternative short-term treatment. Helped by a small viewing telescope, the surgeon can clear your hip-joint of loose particles and trim down irregular surfaces, so relieving the pain of arthritis. The operation is minimally invasive, so that no stitches are required, and patients need stay only a night or two in hospital. What is more, this treatment still allows a THR to be performed at a later stage.

Finally, there are a number of surgical treatments, some extremely radical, available in special cases. Forage, excision arthroplasty, arthrodesis and osteotomy belong to this class, and are alternatives to THR. Because none of them have the advantages of THR, these procedures are not common. To learn more, read Richard Villar's *Hip Replacement: A Patient's Guide to Surgery and Recovery*, which presents a leading surgeon's advice relating to these special cases.

Alternative Medicine

There is no doubting the popularity of alternative medicine, so it is not surprising that it offers quite a number of different treatments for arthritis. In the context of THR, alternative treatment inevitably falls short of the results that the operation achieves. Nothing that it offers will implant a prosthesis, which is what THR is all about. Nor is there much hope of restoring cartilage or other tissue that has worn away with the passing of the years. On the other hand, to you the patient, arthritis of the hip is mainly about suffering, and its effect on the quality of your life. If, then, some alternative treatment reduces your suffering, this may be all you need – or at least think you need, which in the present context is much the same. In the cases described in Chapter 7 where the operative risk is high, it may even be the best treatment available to you.

Homeopathy

Judging by the number of doctors who adopt it, homeopathy is the most respectable form of alternative medicine. It is even accepted by the NHS, when it is adopted by a qualified physician. The focus of homeopathy is you, the patient, rather than your complaint. Treatment is in the form of pills, ointments, lotions, etc., which you can administer yourself, in the same way as most prescription drugs obtained from a chemist. Because homeopathic drugs are free of the disagreeable side-effects that are often a counter-indication for standard medicines, you will probably find them less threatening.

The object of homeopathic medicines is to stimulate the body's self-healing powers. The underlying principle is that once a substance has been identified with a particular ailment, a small but potent dose of the same substance will bring about a cure. In practice this means a choice of natural organic remedies, some of which are claimed to be specific for arthritis. Examples are poison ivy, white or common briony and rue. Practitioners also tend to insist on a modified lifestyle, with little room not only for tobacco and alcohol, but also for tea, coffee, colas, perfume and even household cleaning materials. This may well be more help than the homeopathic specifics.

Acupuncture

Acupuncture is a quite different form of treatment, particularly as it is experienced by the patient. Practitioners treat more arthritis than any other condition. Although treatment can do no more than relieve pain, it may do this more effectively than any alternative. In this case there is a possible physiological explanation. Acupuncture may increase the level of endorphins – chemical compounds occurring naturally in the brain – which are responsible for sensations of pleasure. It may have the same effect on serotonin, a neurotransmitter, whose level in the brain is another measure of well-being. In China, where acupuncture originated, it is used as an anaesthetic for surgery. (I have not come across any case of it being used for a THR.) Once again, everything depends upon the patient.

Acupuncture's underlying principle is that certain specific influences require unobstructed passage through each of the twelve organic systems attributed to the human body. The actual passage is along twelve meridians, which link recognized sensitive points on the skin and connect them with specific organs: these are classified according to which certain specific functions they relate to.

One terminal point of a meridian is always in the head or chest, while the other is in either a hand or a foot. The acupuncture points, which number several hundred, are located at precisely known points along the meridians. Diagnosis consists of selecting the points which are critical for the relevant condition; treatment then involves inserting fine needles into the selected points, to a depth of a few millimetres. Modern practitioners sometimes apply an electric current.

T'ai Chi and Yoga

T'ai Chi and Yoga are part of what alternative medicine has to offer in place of physiotherapy. T'ai Chi is a very distinctive form of exercise that can now be observed in almost any part of the world.

> T'ai Chi is said to have originated when a thirteenth-century Taoist monk, Chang San Feng, observed a fight between a snake and a crane.

Many people without any Chinese ancestry have now adopted T'ai Chi. It consists of adopting a succession of the 108 different postures established by tradition, each one being maintained for several minutes. Since practitioners have no qualms about performing in public, they are commonly seen in parks and other open spaces.

T'ai Chi can be practised just as effectively at home, where with the help of a trained T'ai Chi therapist, you should discover the particular postures that help your condition. You should practise these several times a day. This may be somewhat time-consuming, but the relief of pain and an improved sense of well-being should make it worthwhile.

Yoga, which originated in India, comprises a variety of physical and contemplative exercises designed to liberate the individual from involvement with the material world. Since this is characterized by suffering, it is not surprising that Yoga-based exercises have been developed to counteract the pain of arthritis. The exercises, accompanied by special breathing, are designed to teach sufferers to use their joints in a relaxed way.

Manipulative and Spa Treatments

Another part of what alternative medicine has to offer in place of physiotherapy consists of various forms of hands-on treatment by a trained therapist. Massage, which is also part of clinical physiotherapy, is the most general form: for the patient it involves kneading and stroking different parts of your body. This is a very ancient form of medicine, characterized by the healing coming from a 'laying on of hands', often combined with applying aromatic oils. You will find that the movement of the therapist's hands can take a number of forms – tapping, squeezing, stroking, brushing, vibrating and so on.

Massage is often an adjunct to some form of water therapy, as commonly applied in spas, which may have special hydrotherapy pools for arthritis sufferers. It is important that the water, often warm, comes from natural springs, each with its distinctive chemistry. In a number of European countries such treatment is covered by health insurance. Not surprisingly, the spas, mostly in beautiful locations, are a major part of local service economies.

If, then, you are waiting for a THR in the United Kingdom, you could try a holiday in one of the numerous European spas and find at least temporary relief for your suffering. Budapest is also famous for its baths fed by warm springs, which are to be found in many different parts of the city. It may even be that the NHS is bound by a recent decision of the European Court (see also page 163) to fund such treatment, but I would not advise any British patient to count on it.

Osteopaths and chiropractors offer you manipulative treatment for arthritis, bringing relief from pain and restoring function and mobility to your affected limbs. The technique is more vigorous than simple massage, involving pulling and pushing muscles, which during the session itself can be quite painful. The rest, invariably prescribed to follow the session, should then lead to substantial improvement in your condition.

Aromatherapy and Colour Therapy

If you would like to try some more exotic treatment you could go for aromatherapy or colour therapy. The former is based on oils and essences extracted from a great variety of plants: coriander, cypress, juniper, lemon, pine . . . the list is extensive. Colour therapy is intended to achieve the right balance between the colours comprising your aura. The colour diagnosis made by the therapist will determine your dominant colour, which should then be chosen for clothes and decor within the home. In addition, contact therapy is used to channel the right combination of colours to the patient, with yellow being particularly helpful for arthritis.

3
John Charnley and the Development of THR

When it comes to your own THR, you will understand the operation better if you know something about the way it developed. The idea is simple enough: if you suffer the pain of arthritis in one of your hips, replacing the joint with an implant must cure the condition. The contact surfaces of an artificial joint, whatever they are made of, will not be connected to your sensory nervous system – and no nerves means no pain. The solution to the problem seems obvious, and it is not surprising that the first attempts at solving it in this way go back to the late nineteenth century. Unfortunately, the cure – at least in the long term – was always worse than the disease, or at least that is the way things were until John Charnley, a Lancashire man, began to tackle the problem. This was some time around the middle of the twentieth century – that is, in the lifetime of the majority of today's THR patients, wherever they may happen to be.

As the story unfolds, you will find that the reason why John Charnley succeeded, where others failed, was simple. Charnley concentrated on the properties required by a successful prosthesis. These were twofold: low friction between the contact surfaces and durability after implantation. The Charnley prosthesis solved these problems as none had done beforehand: it is still likely to be the model for the implant you will get for your own THR.

Training to be a Surgeon

John Charnley (1911–82), after being the top scientist at school, went on to study medicine at the University of Manchester in 1929, winning medals, prizes and scholarships, particularly in anatomy and physiology. On the long path to qualifying as a consultant, he passed every examination at the earliest possible moment, so that after only three years' study he graduated both as a physician and a surgeon. This young man was plainly in a hurry, becoming a fully qualified FRCS (Fellow of the Royal College of Surgeons) only four months after his twenty-fifth birthday – the minimum age.

In 1939, aged only twenty-eight, he was appointed the Resident Casualty Officer at the Manchester Royal Infirmary, where, for the first time, he could specialize in orthopaedics. Then, with World War II, Charnley became an officer in the Royal Army Medical Corps. In 1940, he started working in hospitals behind the lines, mainly in Egypt and Palestine.

In 1942, Charnley set up his own orthopaedic workshop, where in collaboration with army engineers (REME) he designed many of the surgical instruments he needed, thus establishing a practice that would continue for the rest of his working life.

Cold Orthopaedics

Once the war was over, Charnley was appointed Resident Surgeon at the Shropshire Orthopaedic Hospital in Oswestry. This was a turning point in his life, for the object was to learn 'cold' orthopaedics – part of what is now called elective surgery. In 1946, traditional orthopaedics was largely concerned with the treatment of bone and joint tuberculosis and the reconstructive surgery needed by polio sufferers. Trauma, mostly in the form of fractures, belonged to general surgery. In the 1950s, effective cures for both TB and polio put an end to traditional orthopaedics and surgeons began to work on the effective surgical treatment of arthritis.

In 1948, Charnley, after only six months at Oswestry, returned to Manchester to become an NHS consultant. The way was open to him to become a leader in his field, which now extended to the surgical treatment of fractures – particularly of the hip.

This, then, is the man to whom you will owe your new

hip prosthesis and, with reasonably good fortune, complete relief from your painful arthritis. Charnley is important, above all, for paying unprecedented attention to the mechanical requirements of surgery. In his Manchester workshop he made such things as the stainless steel screws he required for the fixation of fractures of the neck of the femur (where it is part of the hip-joint).

Low Friction Arthroplasty

Critically for the history of orthopaedics, Charnley began to investigate the lubrication of joints. He already contemplated new surgery that would preserve their function. The end of the road would be THR, or total hip replacement. Charnley himself always referred to this operation as LFA, short for low-friction arthroplasty.

In a pilot centre in the Wrightington Hospital just outside Manchester, which he set up in 1958, Charnley focused on LFA in the context of hip surgery. The surgical remodelling of a diseased joint is known as arthroplasty. There are a number of types, one of which is to replace one, or both, of the joint surfaces, by a prosthesis (as described in Chapter 7). Ideally this procedure not only eliminates the pain caused by an arthritic joint, but also replaces the joint by one free of the conditions that caused the arthritis in the first place.

Modern arthroplasty goes back to 1938, when P.W. Wiles, in London, replaced not only the femoral crown but also the acetabulum, the part of the pelvis into which it fits. Both components were made of stainless steel and fixed to the bones by screws. This, then, was the first THR: the new artificial joint consisted of a ball and socket (based on well-established engineering models) and this became the standard form – as it still is.

Hip replacements continued to be carried out on a small scale, with new materials such as acrylic being used in the prostheses, but although many patients obtained immediate relief, it never lasted more than a few years. So unsatisfactory were the long-term results that Charnley, in 1956, stated that arthroplasty of the hip was 'doomed to failure if only because of the coefficients of friction involved between metal or acrylic material on the one hand, and bone or cartilage on the other'. This conclusion was born out of Charnley's own experience, for he had himself carried out THRs at the end of the 1940s, but with little success. In the 1960s, encouraged by colleagues in other hospitals, he looked anew at this operation in its relation to the anatomy of the hip.

The hip-joint (illustrated in Figure 3) is a synovial joint, in which the contact surface of both the femur and the pelvis is covered with cartilage, a semi-opaque grey or white substance capable of withstanding high pressure. The joint itself is enclosed in a capsule, filled with *synovial* fluid. Arthritis occurs when the cartilage is worn away, so that the two bones comprising a joint are in direct contact. In 1960 orthopaedic surgeons believed that the imperfect fit of the crown of the femur into the

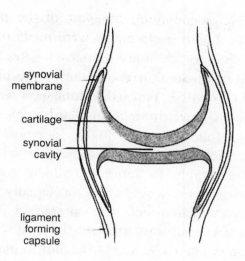

synovial
membrane

cartilage

synovial
cavity

ligament
forming
capsule

Figure 3
A synovial joint

acetabulum made it essential for the joint to be lubri-cated by the synovial fluid.

After consulting colleagues from the engineering department of Manchester University, Charnley became convinced that this view was incorrect, largely because movements of the joint are relatively slow. At the same time, cartilage is resilient, so that the contact surfaces of the two bones comprising a joint will be substantial, whatever their position in any state of motion.

The alternative is boundary lubrication, which relies on very low levels of friction between sliding surfaces – such as in skiing. This is what is important for a joint, whether natural or artificial, since its function is to allow the two bones defining it to move relative to each other.

Charnley's problem was to measure the degree of

friction in human joints. Here he discovered that an obscure Dr Jones, in the course of the 1930s, had done just this, but for the knee-joints of horses. Dr Jones, following on the work of the seventeenth-century Dutch scientist Christiaan Huygens, developed a pendulum system to measure the friction in a horse's knee-joint. Charnley, following Dr Jones, designed his own apparatus, which he used to show that synovial fluid was quite unable to lubricate human joints at all adequately. They would operate equally effectively when dry, which in one way simplified the task of designing a workable prosthesis.

Still, the problem remained of finding materials, A and B, for the artifical joint in the prosthesis, with the friction between them at a sufficiently low level. Experiments showed that with the materials then used in prostheses, the level of friction was nowhere near good enough. No wonder, then, that none of the THRs carried out in the 1950s were successful in the long term. If, however, the other surface was cartilage, the lower figure could be achieved.

The nub of the problem is that the object of THR is to deal with hips where there is little, if any, cartilage present – which (as shown in Chapter 1) is why those with this condition suffer from arthritis. This explains why Charnley, from some time late in the 1950s, set his sights on low-friction arthroplasty. In 1958, he decided that 'the only chance of success in lubricating an artificial joint would be by using surfaces which were inherently slippery on each other'. By this time Charnley had discovered that a hemi-arthroplasty, with only the crown of the femur being replaced, was not satisfactory, at least when – to give it greater strength – the prosthesis was made of metal.

Charnley again looked for help outside the world of medicine. The quest led to a plastic known in the trade as polytetrafluorethylene (PTFE), but to the general public as Teflon. The prosthesis consisted of a thin shell shaped to cover the head of the femur, fitting into a lining of the acetabulum made of the same material. This combination made for unprecedented mobility of the hip combined with complete relief of pain – at least during the months directly following the LFA operation.

Charnley was not satisfied, largely because the PTFE cap fitted to the femur was likely to damage the blood supply to the bone. He decided to discard the cap and instead fit a metallic prosthesis. The spherical head of the new prosthesis was attached to a long stem, to be implanted inside the femur – requiring the surgery described in Chapter 5. This new technique then confronted Charnley with the problem of finding a suitable cement, to secure the stem of the prosthesis inside the femur.

A New Prosthesis

At much the same time, Charnley's engineering colleagues persuaded him to make a radical change in the design of the prosthesis. Orthopaedic surgeons had always accepted that the size of the two sides to the artificial joint should be much the same as that of a natural hip-joint. The result was that the diameter of the ball and socket was

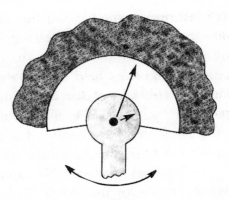

Figure 4
The fit of a Charnley prothesis with a small femoral head

about 42 mm – approximately that of a golf ball. According to best engineering practice, the diameter should be reduced to the smallest possible value at which the prosthesis would still carry the expected load.

The final stage, reached after a process of trial and error across several LFA operations, was a diameter of 22.25 mm, little more than half that of almost any earlier prosthesis. First, the contact surface would be much smaller, allowing a substantial reduction in friction; second, a much more substantial socket could be implanted in the acetabulum. The main disadvantage is that with a smaller diameter, the risk of dislocation – a major hazard with THR – is increased. The optimal size depends upon a trade-off between positive and negative factors.

Although Charnley first started to develop LFA in the 1950s, it was not until the early 1970s that the final stage was reached, with a prosthesis which could be relied upon to last indefinitely. To begin with he saw his operation as a last resort, suitable only for 'subjects with the poor muscles and relatively feeble morale which so often accompany long-continued ill-health and old age'. From this perspective, once a satisfactory prosthesis had been developed, it could be reckoned upon to last the life of the patient.

At this early stage, Charnley's mind-set was hardly optimistic, and he readily stated his belief that 'in joint surgery . . . mobility and stability are incompatible' – a statement which would astonish most of the hundreds of thousands of patients who have now had his operation. Although he made remarkable progress throughout the 1960s, all was not plain sailing.

Sometime in 1962 it became clear that Teflon was nowhere near as good a material for prostheses as had been thought. Quite simply it was not strong enough, so that in the course of time wear and tear produced small granular particles, which then coalesced in a sort of cheesy material surrounding the joint. The prosthesis, reduced in size, no longer had the required tight fit in the joint, so that the hip became painful – the very symptom that the operation was designed to cure. The immediate result was that Charnley felt himself committed to perform revision operations for all the patients who suffered in this way. At the same time, it was clear that Teflon could no longer be used in prostheses.

HMWP – A New Material

Then, in the summer of 1962, chance led to the discovery of a new material that was much harder wearing than Teflon. In this way, HMWP – high molecular weight polyethylene – became the standard material for the cup to be fitted into the acetabulum. It had some disadvantages, such as a somewhat higher degree of friction, but these were far outweighed by its durability.

Following all the trouble he had had with Teflon, Charnley was extremely cautious in his use of HMWP, operating only on patients over sixty-eight years old, who were extremely disabled.

At this stage also, Charnley was extremely guarded in allowing other surgeons to carry out LFA operations. He saw to it that his design of prostheses could only be supplied to surgeons he had himself approved, and such approval was only granted to those who had attended a short course at Wrightington. This was not a way to make friends in the profession, and in April 1968, Charnley wrote:

> I realize that the snowballing effect of the operation is getting out of hand, and with the passage of time and the accumulation of experience, my views are now being forced into a different line from the extremely cautious and rather obstructive attitude which I have taken heretofore . . . the time had now come to declare that this procedure has been tested for five years in the human body and can now be fully developed.

Even so, Charnley was still not very forthcoming, and it was not until the 1970s that the LFA operation was open to any surgeon who wished to carry it out.

Although this marks the time at which LFA became a standard procedure, worldwide, for treating arthritis of the hip, the 1960s witnessed quite a number of new prostheses, which were variants developed by surgeons who had visited Charnley and exchanged information with him. Nonetheless, Charnley's technique and the prosthesis he developed became definitive in the field of THR.

The year 1970 marks the breakthrough on to the world scene. In this year Charnley published his key paper, 'Total hip replacement by low friction arthroplasty' and two years later another paper, 'The long-term results of low friction arthroplasty of the hip performed as a primary intervention' assessed the results of the operation.

Cement and Clean Air

The success of LFA depended on two factors to which Charnley devoted much time and energy: the first was the development of the right cement for fixing the prosthesis on one side in the medulla, or hollow shaft, of the femur, and on the other, in the acetabulum. The second factor was the need to ensure clean air in the operating theatre so as to guard against bacterial infection. Given that this is a quite general problem in major surgery (dealt with in Chapter 5), Charnley's somewhat idiosyncratic solutions are marginal to his lifetime's dedication to LFA. His commitment to finding the right cement is, however, central to it.

Charnley always accepted that there could be no

perfect fit for the prosthesis, whether in the femur or the acetabulum. To provide the necessary space for the prosthesis to be inserted, both had to be 'reamed' – that is, shaped by surgical means to a form that would admit the prosthesis. For Charnley there was never any question of achieving a tight fit that would be sufficient to ensure long-term stability. This meant that a cement had to be used to ensure a stable implant.

Charnley first confronted the problem in the late 1950s, when he was using prostheses to repair fractures of the upper femur. Borrowing from the experience of dentists, he chose to work with a self-curing acrylic cement, prepared by mixing a powder with a fluid in a bowl. The scene is reminiscent of a kitchen rather than a workshop: the mixture first becomes creamy, then doughy and after three or four minutes it begins to set. At this stage it is rammed into the medulla of the femur, and the prosthesis hammered in. In the process, the dough is forced into every crevice of the femur and, as it sets, the prosthesis is anchored firmly inside the medulla. To help counter bacterial infection, Charnley sterilized the powder directly before the operation; he also added barium-sulphate so that after the operation the cement would show up on X-ray photographs.

Charnley died in 1982, just short of his seventieth birthday. He was then younger than most of the patients he thought suitable for THR. To the end of his life he gave older people priority when it came to an operation. Once, at a congress in Las Vegas, his advice was asked in the case of a young woman. After looking at X-ray photographs of her hips, his answer was the single word, 'aspirin'. He would not have dared say that today.

It was not only on the question of age that Charnley remained remarkably conservative. The fact that he always stuck to stainless steel for the shaft of the prosthesis, without seriously considering the advantages of titanium or a chrome-cobalt alloy as alternatives, suggests a reluctance to move with the times. By today's standards he also seems ultra-cautious, as for instance in his insistence on patients walking with a stick for the first six weeks after the operation. He was also reluctant to prescribe anticoagulants, finding that the increased risk of bleeding outweighed the prevention of pulmonary embolisms – a considerable risk when it comes to major orthopaedic operations such as THR.

Although Charnley died just over twenty years ago, the scope for THR and the number of operations carried out have increased enormously. Younger patients are now commonly accepted, with the prosthesis being implanted uncemented, as explained in Chapter 7. THR is a routine operation within the competence of any orthopaedic surgeon. Indeed, in a teaching hospital, a patient is more than likely to be operated on by a trainee house surgeon. In the last year of his life, Charnley accepted that the operation was 'deceptively easy to perform' but emphasized that the success rate was much higher with trained specialist surgeons.

The Charnley Hip

There is no doubt that John Charnley had few equals among his contemporaries in orthopaedic surgery. An editorial in the *British Medical Journal*, published five years after his death, explains why his work was so important:

> Despite the Charnley hip being one of the first joints to be used in large numbers twenty-five years ago, it still reigns supreme – the gold standard. Not one of the dozens of newer more expensive implants being used by surgeons can match the figures obtained with the Charnley hip in skilled hands.

Charnley stands out not only as a very gifted surgeon whose skills were immediately apparent to colleagues who saw him operate, but also as a professional man who worked willingly with specialists in other fields, particularly engineering. His passionate interest in mechanical systems was critical to his success in solving the technical problems of joint replacement. The key innovation was the drastic reduction in the diameter of the head of the femoral prosthesis and of the acetabulum cap into which it fitted. This reduced the friction to a level comparable to that of a natural joint.

At the same time, Charnley, after much trial and error, found all the right materials, whether for the cement, the metal in the femoral prosthesis or the plastic in the acetabulum cup. Although, in response to the demands from surgeons in different parts of the world, the medical supply industry continues to provide any number of alternatives, Charnley's hip is still the standard by which they are measured. The improvements – if such they are – made since his death are small in comparison to what he achieved in the last twenty-five years of his life.

Now, in the twenty-first century, Charnley's low friction arthroplasty relieves hundreds of thousands of patients every year, in every part of the world, of the agonies of arthritis in the hip. I know, because I speak from my own experience.

4
The Time Factor

The First Symptoms

Time, both actual and potential, is always problematic for THR patients, as you will soon discover. To begin with you have the problem of recognizing the first symptoms, as described in Chapter 1, and being sufficiently concerned about them to consult your GP. By manipulating and examining your leg on the afflicted side, he will make a first assessment of loss of function and mobility, helped by your description of the pain you suffer and your level of disability. If, then, the symptoms indicate arthritis of the hip, you will almost certainly be referred to a hospital for X-rays. These will show whether, and to what extent, cartilage is worn away at the afflicted joint. Other abnormalities associated with the condition may also be apparent.

At this stage your GP may well recommend waiting, with periodic check-ups. The arthritis can progress very slowly, and given that a hip prosthesis does not last for ever, there are definite advantages – already noted in Chapter 3 – in postponing an operation. The main disadvantage, however, is in the length of hospital waiting lists for THRs.

The result is that if, to begin with, you delay taking further action, when the pain and discomfort become more acute you are likely to have to wait months for surgery. In spite of recent government promises to reduce the period of waiting for NHS patients to a maximum of six months, it is by no means certain that this can be done. And even six months can be a long time if you suffer from arthritis of the hip. I would advise you, therefore, to ask for a referral to an orthopaedic surgeon at a relatively early stage.

The request for a hospital appointment will confront you with the next waiting period. You will wait some weeks for your consultation with the orthopaedic surgeon, and it is only then that your name can be put on the waiting list for surgery. Your GP, by shopping around, may be able to help in finding the local hospital with the shortest waiting time for the first consultation, but this is only the first round. The same hospital may prove to have much longer waiting times for the actual operation. It may be possible to discover, with the very first telephone call, whether this is the case.

At this stage it is helpful to know something of the problem of time and space in hospital organization, and its relationship to the personnel – medical and otherwise – who will be dealing with you. The basic unit is the department, which in the present case will be orthopaedic surgery. Its size will vary from one hospital to another, and there are even specialist orthopaedic hospitals such as the Royal National Orthopaedic Hospital in Stanmore, on the outskirts of London. The trend is towards larger units, with the advantages of economies of scale and specialist surgeons whose work is largely confined to joint replacement.

The size of the department will be defined by the number of specialist consultants, the number of beds they dispose of, and the facilities available to them. In orthopaedics the key facility is the operating theatre, of which there will be several available in a typical large modern hospital. In small hospitals, they may have to be shared with other surgical departments, which may affect waiting lists.

Supporting services, such as X-rays, blood-testing, supply of medicines and physiotherapy, each with its own niche in the hospital organization, are provided centrally. You will get to know them all soon enough.

What counts for you, as a THR patient, is the number of specialists qualified to carry out the operation. There is a whole hierarchy in British hospitals, with consultants at the top, followed by registrars and so on down the line, but routine THRs may well be carried out by a trainee surgeon, under the supervision of a consultant. In a large teaching hospital, you may see little of the consultant in charge of your case, but at the end of the day, it is the consultants who call the shots.

Traditionally it is the number of beds that the consultants dispose of in the department that decides their overall strategy when it comes to planning operations.

This is now changing with the trend towards much shorter stays in hospital, with an increasing number of operations – though not, so far, THRs – being carried out from out-patient or day-care departments. (Thirty years ago John Charnley reckoned on his patients remaining five weeks in hospital: after my THR at the end of 2001, I was discharged after only five days.)

A sufficient number of orthopaedic beds is only half the problem, particularly with elective surgery such as THR. Operating theatres are another possible bottleneck. State-of-the-art equipment, particularly for anesthesia, is very expensive, and there must be specially trained nursing staff. In this case, good planning makes all the difference in the efficient use of resources: where one hospital fits in only three operations in a day, another will fit in twice as many. Here the most efficient strategy is to book a theatre for a whole day devoted to one type of operation, say THR.

The Orthopaedic Surgeon's Practice

The many different kinds of operation required of orthopaedic surgeons means that the above is easier said than done. Because this factor directly affects the waiting list for THRs, the working life of the orthopaedic surgeon must be looked at more closely. Once again, it is useful to remember that orthopaedics is that branch of medicine concerned with correcting deformities in or repairing damage to the muscular-skeletal system: its focus is on the surgery of bones and joints, as is shown by the title of the *Journal of Bone and Joint Surgery*, its principal medical journal.

The domain of orthopaedics falls naturally into two main areas: correcting deformities such as arthritis of the hip, and treating bone fractures and dislocations (at the same time repairing the accompanying damage to other tissue). The first area is part of elective surgery: the patient must take some initiative in setting up the operation. The second area is within the realm of traumatology – trauma being the general medical term for injury. Although this may be psychological as well as physical, only the latter is in the realm of orthopaedic surgery.

When it comes to patients listed for elective surgery, of which you will be one, a hospital orthopaedic department has at any given time a fairly precise long-term view of the task in front of it. Basically, you and all the other patients in line for surgery will be known for a long time, being kept on a waiting list in the computer system according to various criteria defining your respective priorities. The basic principle can be taken to be 'first come, first served', as long as it is recognized that the consultants who run the department have the right to define some cases as more urgent than others.

I would not advise you to accuse another patient of queue-jumping. In any hospital the consultant's word is law on a matter of this kind. In principle, the list for up to a month from any given date should be more or less firm, but it can happen that you will be called up for a THR at no more than 24 hours' notice. (Your operation could also be cancelled at 24 hours' notice.) Where there is a long waiting list, months can pass without your hearing anything until you are suddenly called up for surgery. Occasional telephone calls to the department secretary (particularly if coming from your GP) may help find out how things are going, but this cannot be counted on.

Trauma

The uncertainty relating to waiting lists for THRs and other elective orthopaedic surgery is compounded by the need for the surgeons to spend a substantial part of their time dealing with trauma. Trauma patients tend to be admitted via the Accident and Emergency Department of the hospital: in principle, the first consultation, with one of the doctors on duty, should take place without delay, and this will certainly be the case where there is serious injury requiring immediate treatment if the life of the patient is to be saved. (Of course anyone looking at the TV news will know about trolley-patients, who may well be trauma cases.)

In practice, really urgent cases (some of which will require one of the intensive care beds allocated to orthopaedics) are the exception rather than the rule. Most fractures seen by the doctors in A and E are referred, after what is essentially first aid, to a consultation several days later in the orthopaedic outpatients section – which may take the form of a special fracture clinic. However this may be, the consultant surgeon may recommend conservative, rather than intrusive treatment, so that, for example, the site of the fracture will be encased in fibreglass plaster. This is the job of a paramedic, and the consultant will hardly be involved further.

On the other hand, the consultant may decide on surgery, in which case the date, mostly a day or two later, will be booked on the spot, with immediate admission to a ward. A moment's thought will show that trauma surgery introduces considerable uncertainty into the working life of the orthopaedic surgeon. On a typical Monday morning he will not know what operations, on which trauma patients, he will be carrying out before the end of the week. This is true even when many of these patients will already have been seen by the doctors in A and E.

In practice, the need to treat trauma patients follows a rule of statistical averages, with regular fluctuations, so that football injuries – the bane of many orthopaedic surgeons – are known to peak in March and September, while road accidents are at their worst on winter and bank holiday weekends, particularly when the weather is bad. The problem is that the choice between conservative or operative treatment is likely to be influenced not only by such factors, but also by the mind-set of each individual surgeon within the department. On a Monday morning, the surgeon dealing with out-patients might send a patient with a broken ankle to a ward, to await surgery later in the week; a day later, a colleague might send the same patient to have the bone set in a cast, to then be sent home with crutches.

A hospital orthopaedic department generally knows only too well where the different surgeons stand when it comes to the choice between conservative and operative treatment of trauma, but no one will give this away to the patient (although you may discover this for yourself). The point is that an orthopaedic department may have more freedom than it cares to admit when it comes to striking a balance between trauma patients and those waiting for elective surgery.

Ideally, the two should be dealt with separately, so that the two classes of patient do not even share the same wards (which would also help protect THR patients against bacterial infection spreading from the wounds of trauma patients.) It is perfectly possible for fixed days to be set aside for the use of operating theatres for elective surgery, particularly the fitting of prostheses. Where there's a will, there's a way, is the principle that should govern here, and to be fair, some NHS hospitals have applied it successfully in keeping down waiting lists for elective surgery such as THR.

Elective Surgery

Some consultants confine their practice to elective surgery. This has obvious benefits for patients, but in practice these are more likely to be found outside the NHS – a topic dealt with in Chapter 10.

In other cases, however, an orthopaedic department can allow trauma patients to swamp those waiting for elective surgery, simply on the basis that operations carried out on the former allow for little or no delay. In medical terms, the pathology defines the timetable in traumatology. There are, however, so many variables which count when it comes to allocating a hospital's surgical resources, whether human or material, that sub-optimal use is too often the order of the day. This is particularly likely to be the case where there is every incentive to accept the status quo, as in the NHS. Sadly, also, for those waiting for a THR, trauma patients have a much higher profile: this is not just true of David Beckham, but of any teenage footballer with a similar injury. Who knows, but a few more red cards might help cut waiting lists for THRs.

THRs and the Bottom Line

All this leaves you, and other THR patients, pretty helpless, with 'grin and bear it' the order of the day. You are not without friends, however: your condition has been discovered as a useful stick with which to beat the NHS. The government got the message, and set up targets for many kinds of surgery, including THR. Now targets appear to be counter-productive, and it is still uncertain whether the promise to cut waiting lists to six months will be kept.

Everything turns on money, so it is not surprising that the first step is to increase the level of NHS contributions. More money will certainly pay for training more orthopaedic surgeons, but it does not necessarily mean that sufficient young men and women will opt for this particular career (although recent trends point in this direction). It takes ten years or more to qualify, however, so this is hardly a short-term solution.

There is, in any case, a race against time. Whatever the failings of the NHS, in the generation following John Charnley's successes, it has had to find the means to offer an entirely new operation to tens of thousands of patients every year.

Taking seventy as the median age for THR patients, the percentage of the UK population above that age is substantially higher than it was a generation ago, when today's standard operation was first introduced.

The much greater demand for THRs is no news. We all know about the ageing population. It is still something of a miracle that the NHS has coped at all, particularly when most of you who are waiting to be operated on are

> The cost to the NHS of a THR is at the level of the standard UK old age pension for a whole year. Multiplied by 50,000, this is very big money.

of pensionable age, and therefore pay no contribution to the cost of the health services provided for you.

When the NHS has really got its act together on THRs – if that day ever comes – some 10 per cent of the population of pensionable age, with women outnumbering men two to one, will sooner or later have the benefit of this operation, some more than once.

The Orthopaedic Surgeon's Workload

All this must be looked at in terms of the total workload of orthopaedic surgeons in relation to the numbers of THRs they carry out. According to the latest figures, relating to 2000–2001, each of 1,148 orthopaedic surgeons performs on average 711 operations a year within the NHS. Of these, about 6 per cent will be THRs, with about the same number of knee prosthesis implants. This means that within the NHS the average surgeon performs less than fifty THRs in a year: this may sound unimpressive, but allowing to each such operation two hours of theatre time, the surgeon would devote two full working weeks to THRs.

Another two hours per patient could well be needed for consultations both before and after the operation, ward visits during the period of your admission and all the background administration required to deal with your case. Many surgeons also spend a week or two every year attending specialist conferences, critically important for keeping up with the latest state-of-the-art research and practice.

To get the right perspective, it is essential to realise that a THR is a major operation. Orthopaedic surgery can be much simpler: common minor operations, such as those that remedy carpal tunnel syndrome, can take about ten minutes, and are performed on out-patients. It follows that less than half of the 700-odd operations that a surgeon performs in a year require the full range of hospital services, including admission to a surgical ward. Probably some 10 per cent of the operations performed take up more than 50 per cent of a surgeon's time (and THRs fall within this category).

It is not all that odd, then, that a surgeon must devote up to two weeks of his time to just fifty THRs. In practice, many surgeons do better than this, and a rate of 150 THRs a year is not unknown in a general orthopaedic department. There are also surgeons who perform few, if any, THRs, and the trend is towards concentration, so that only a minority of surgeons have a significant THR practice. The handful of specialists who do nothing but hip surgery perform up to 600 THRs a year (and John Charnley was up to performing nine in a single day). At this level, however, most of the operations will be outside the NHS (and so are not counted in the figures given above).

In the last fifteen years, the number of orthopaedic surgeons working in the NHS has increased by more than 70 per cent, but many will have a private practice on the side. This may explain why there has been no comparable increase in productivity, measured according to the number of THR operations performed in a year. This is discouraging when it comes to assessing the government's latest plans for increased spending on the NHS, particularly when the present figure of 50,000 THRs performed in a year is likely to increase to a much higher level. If, then, waiting lists are brought down everywhere to under six months, this will be a remarkable achievement.

Shopping Around for Treatment

What hope does all this offer to you as you wait for a THR? Are the government's present plans nothing more than spin? Time will tell. Nonetheless, with new freedom to shop around different hospitals, you can do something to improve your lot. There will, however, be a price to pay. According to a recent survey among THR patients, only 5 per cent would accept treatment in a hospital 30 miles away from home, even if that saved months on the waiting list.

Here I can speak from my own experience. The first hospital I went to for a consultation had a waiting list not far short of a year. A large teaching hospital with a first-class reputation – particularly in orthopaedics – it was just within walking distance of my home (though not for hip patients).

I thought I could do better. After shopping around, on and off the Web, I found a provincial hospital some fifty miles away, with waiting times of less than a month. The head of the orthopaedic department had trained under John Charnley and much preferred prosthesis implants – including THRs – to dealing with trauma. He set fixed days apart for such operations, and worked with a specially trained team. Mine was the first of six operations in one day. No wonder that his hospital had no waiting lists for THRs.

Both the nursing staff, and the other patients on the ward, were amazed – in a friendly sort of way – that I had found it worthwhile to travel fifty miles for my operation, and I was rather a fish out of water.

In the world of modern surgery it is easy to find scape-
goats, particularly in the UK where people, egged on by
the media, seem to enjoy bashing the NHS. The NHS
certainly has its faults, as we all know only too well, but
you might just consider that yours is the first generation,
ever, that could be relieved, by surgery, of a condition
that otherwise would cause you unremitting pain and
distress. Look once again at the case of my old school-
master, Bill Cheesman, described in the Introduction. At
the same time, if you want to get the best out of the
NHS, you should shop around: who knows what you
might find? And if government promises are kept, things
will only get better.

5
Operative Risks

Given the extraordinary success of THR in the field of orthopaedic surgery you will be inclined to overlook the risks inherent in the operation and its aftermath. Since THR is essentially elective, however, you should certainly be aware of the risks it involves, even though they affect only a small minority – about 5 per cent – of patients.

The question of risk tends to be downplayed by doctors, although most will give straight answers to any questions put to them. The truth of the matter has been well stated by a leading American surgeon, Sherwin B. Nuland: 'If there is a single characteristic of medicine that every layperson should be aware of when accepting or rejecting an offered medical procedure, it must certainly be its inherent uncertainty.'

The right perspective is critically important. You, as a THR patient, are more than likely to be relatively old: you may well have passed your seventieth if not your eightieth birthday. At this stage in life, mortality steadily increases, so that, for example, out of every 100,000 men who became seventy in the period 1998–2000, some 3,317 men failed to become seventy-one, while for women, who tend to live longer, the figure was 1,981.

Out of the same 100,000, some 700 men and 1,400 women had a THR in the seventy-first year of their life (although precise figures are not available). Of these, two or three probably did not survive the operation, but it is to be noted that this is a very small figure in relation to the total mortality. Looking at it in another way, on your seventieth birthday, the chance that you will not live another year as a result of a failed THR is less than 0.001 per cent. (The operative risk with, say, a heart double-bypass, is some ten times as great.) If, then, a surgeon (or more likely, an anaesthetist) tells a patient that death as a result of the operation is very improbable, this is the truth. (At the end of the 1960s John Charnley was content with a mortality of 1 per cent: the risk today is substantially less.) All in all, your chance of dying as a result of a THR is almost certainly less than one in 1,000 – but then of course the great majority of people never need a THR in the first place. The figures can be slanted one way or another, but even so, the risk factor with a THR compared with other major surgery is very small. Acquainting you with the major risks, however small, is the purpose of this chapter.

Your medical history is a key factor when it comes to risk. Before the operation, the anaesthetist will look at this very closely, and will be particularly interested in any previous operations you may have had. Cardiac and respiratory problems, obesity, diabetes and any number of other conditions increase the risk inherent in major surgery. In the specific case of THR, bone conditions such as osteoporosis are inevitably a relevant risk factor.

Your relatively advanced age significantly increases the probability that one or more of these conditions form part of your medical history. Plainly, in such cases the operative risk is higher, to the point that in an extreme case your surgery may have to be postponed, if not cancelled altogether.

When all is said and done, well over 99 per cent of all patients survive the operation itself. Even so, as you lie in the recovery room, you are not quite out of the woods. Things can still go wrong as a result of risks that are not life-threatening. First, it may become apparent that either the sciatic or the femoral nerve – depending on the surgeon's approach – has been damaged as a result of the operation. If no action is taken, injury to the sciatic nerve may leave you with a club foot, so in such a case, immediate remedial surgery may be necessary. Where the femoral nerve is damaged, the consequences of damage are less drastic.

One common result of a THR is change in the difference between the lengths your legs, although as noted on page 104, the surgeon, by choosing the right components for the prosthesis, can minimize the chances of this happening. At all events, surveys carried out among patients six months after their operation suggest that this factor little affects their satisfaction and comfort, or the function of the new joint.

Bacterial Infection

As with other invasive surgery, the most daunting prospect you face is that of a bacterial infection, which can mean a real trail of sorrows. In the world around us bacteria are present everywhere, in countless different shapes and sizes, not all of them harmful. The skin is the body's main defence against them. This explains why infection by harmful bacteria most commonly comes through the mouth and other parts of the body open to the outside without being protected by skin. A wound, therefore, which exposes internal tissue, constitutes an obvious risk of bacterial infection – something that the medical profession has known since well before the end of the nineteenth century.

The problem with invasive surgery, such as THR, is that your hip-joint can only be reached by inflicting a deep wound, accompanied by substantial loss of blood and considerable exposure of internal tissue. The risk of bacterial infection is then considerable, and hospitals go to endless trouble in ensuring sterile conditions in their operating theatres. Access is closely controlled and those who are admitted are subject to very strict protocols. Medical personnel working within a theatre wear special clothing, with masks and rubber gloves to reduce the chances of their transmitting bacteria to patients being operated on.

At the same time, the air will be filtered and circulated, as far as possible, in a way that will take micro-organisms (of which there will be millions) away from the site of the operation. John Charnley went to extreme lengths to ensure this result, at the cost of the comfort and mobility of the surgeon.

> A good hospital, by adopting all the means available, can reduce the risk of bacterial infection to under 1 per cent, but there is consider-able variation – up to 12 per cent in extreme cases – in the standards actually reached.

Whatever is done to reduce the presence of harmful bacteria in the operating theatre, this may still not be sufficient. The answer is to apply antibiotic drugs to the site of the operation, for instance by mixing them into the cement. This is a standard precaution.

Bacterial infection may well come from your own body. As a result of poor oral hygiene, your teeth may be a source, and you should certainly have a dental check-up shortly before being operated upon, with particular attention being paid to your wisdom teeth – if you still have any. If an extraction is necessary, the risk of infection is so high that two or three weeks should be allowed to pass before any THR. Burns and bladder conditions (just possibly including infection through the catheter inserted after local anaesthesia) are also a source of risk.

A bacterial infection is most likely to occur before you are discharged from hospital, but the risk, although steadily decreasing, remains for as long as two years. The consequences of such infection can be drastic. A new operation may be required to remove the prosthesis, only to replace it after the infection has been successfully treated with antibiotics. This may require several weeks in hospital, with your mobility severely restricted.

Dislocation

Dislocation is the other main risk following a THR. In this case, the responsibility lies mainly with you, the patient. The problem is twofold. First, following the implant of the prosthesis, two or three months are needed before hip function and mobility are fully restored. During this period you must take care not to cross the leg on the operated side over the other leg, nor to bend the upper part of the body so that the angle between it and the thighs is less than 90 degrees.

In particular, the required restrictions determine your position while asleep. For the first two or three months after a THR, you will be advised either to lie on your back or on the operated side of your body, avoiding the foetal position at all costs. This may be something of a counsel of perfection, since very few cases have ever been reported of dislocation occurring to patients lying in bed, and a number of surgeons will now allow you right from the start to sleep in any position you find comfortable. The majority, however, stick to the old rule: better safe than sorry.

Second, because the crown to the stem of the prosthesis, and the cup into which it fits, are substantially smaller than with a natural joint, the chances of dislocation are also increased over the long term. You should therefore plan your life so as to control situations likely to put undue stress on the joint.

My own informal survey among patients recovering from a THR suggests that you should take particular care when travelling by public transport, gardening or pursuing any other activity at ground level. Among my circle of acquaintances, one suffered dislocation as a result of stepping off a bus, and two others while gardening. Be warned. In all possible cases, common sense, combined with an appreciation of the risks involved, is the best guide.

Dislocation is extremely painful and requires immediate attention. The two components in your prosthesis will have to be restored to their proper position, and this may even require surgery – followed by the same long-term recuperation as after a THR.

Deep Vein Thrombosis

Finally, there is the risk of deep vein thrombosis and small pulmonary emboli inherent in almost all orthopaedic surgery. As a result of media publicity, the former has recently become known as 'economy class syndrome'. Although in the reported cases it is almost always fatal, prompt action can, and often does, retrieve the situation. This is just as well, for when you are forced to be immobile as a result of major surgery, you are as much at risk as any economy class air passenger. Hospitals know this, and at the very least will have all the apparatus for emergency treatment on stand-by.

Prevention, however, is better than cure, so you are

likely to be fitted with special DVT stockings. You might also start on a prophylactic course of anticoagulants on the evening before the operation, which will continue as long as the risk remains – which may mean a period of weeks continuing long after discharge from hospital. The problem here is that there are a number of counter-indications, particularly relating to the fact that the blood is thinner as a result of the treatment (particularly hazardous for the very old). Intensive medical supervision, with regular blood tests to control the rate of clotting, is therefore essential, which explains why this procedure is not common in the UK (although it is standard in some other countries). Instead, in the UK you may be given injections while you remain in hospital, and simply told to wear DVT stockings after discharge.

Legal Responsibility

With all the things that can go wrong after a THR operation, it is natural to be concerned, and in the event that something *does* go wrong, to ask questions about legal liability. First, a word of warning: medical negligence is an extremely controversial issue. A fundamental principle in this branch of the law is that you, the patient, consent to the risks inherent in the treatment; the best advice I can offer is for you to ask what these risks are as soon as a THR is advised, and if not then, at some later stage before the operation. This section of the book should suggest to you the right questions to put to the surgeon.

In itself, the fact that medical treatment, including surgery, either fails to produce the results hoped for, or does so at the cost of pathological conditions that make the cure worse than the disease, are seldom if ever sufficient cause for suing those responsible. According a review of 30,000 hospital admissions in New York State, published in 1991 in the *New England Journal of Medicine*. '. . . nearly 4 per cent of hospital patients suffered complications from treatment which prolonged their hospital stay or resulted in disability or death, and that two-thirds of such complications were due to errors in care. One in four, or 1 per cent of admissions, involved actual negligence.' The figure for THRs in the UK is almost certainly much lower.

It follows that there must always be something more than a poor outcome, and the burden will rest upon you to prove that this is the case. Someone on the medical team, not necessarily a doctor or specialist, must have done something that any competent practitioner would have avoided, to cause the damage you complain of. The diffficulty is that what for one specialist falls within a reasonable margin of error, for another falls way outside it. This explains why, in the cases coming before the courts, each side lines up its own team of professional witnesses.

In one example reported in 1991 relating to THRs, the claimant alleged that severe loss of function following over-extension of the sciatic nerve in the process of dislocation described on page 70 was the result of negligence on the part of the surgeon. The claim succeeded, because the court accepted the evidence of the surgeons called as witnesses, that the risk of such damage would have been clearly apparent to a competent practitioner. Steps could, and *should*, have been taken to avoid it.

This case, and many others relating to medical negligence, turned largely on the condition of one particular patient, combined with the relative inexperience of the operating surgeon. In slightly different circumstances the claim could well have failed.

In another case from the mid-1990s, a patient who claimed for pain and suffering as a result of a severe headache in the course of recovery from local anaesthesia had to accept that this was a normal risk: no damages were awarded. Here, there was almost certainly a breakdown of communication – a common factor in medical negligence cases.

Generally, there are very few cases of medical negligence concerning THRs. In 1989 (the last year with complete figures), 34 claims relating to orthopaedic surgery came before the English courts, and few of these related to THRs. Some 70,000 THRs are now carried out every year in the UK (and more than a million in the world as a whole). Less than 5 per cent will lead to the undesirable complications described in this chapter and there will be a much smaller number of deaths. In any one year the number of legal claims for medical negligence, following from such negative outcomes, can then be counted on the fingers of one hand, and most of these will fail.

The message is simple: the THR operation can go wrong, although this does not happen all that often.

This is part of the unavoidable risk with major surgery of this order, and a good surgeon or anaesthetist should make this clear at the start. At the same time, the patient should not hesitate to ask searching questions – even when the specialist is anxious to get on to his next patient.

When it comes to THR, the important point is that bacterial infection, DVT, dislocation and miscellaneous other horrors only occur in a small minority of cases. What is more, when they do occur, they can almost always be treated successfully. The message is simple about any of these possible outcomes: cross that bridge *if and when* you come to it. Instead, as the day comes for your THR, be optimistic and think ahead to how great you will feel when you no longer suffer the pain and discomfort of an arthritic hip.

6

Before the Operation

Preparing the Patient

The treatment provided for a THR patient while waiting for the operation is much the same as that described in the first section of Chapter 2, *Mainline Medical Care*. As, however, the day appointed for surgery comes closer, the treatment will become more focused on preparing the patient for the trauma that this will involve. At the same time, the first steps can be taken to help the process of recovery immediately after the operation.

Patients enjoying good health – who may be the exception rather than the rule in the age groups to which most belong – require little by way of advance preparation. In principle there is no reason why they should be not admitted to hospital on the day of the operation. Although this is normal practice in America, British and continental hospitals generally insist on admission the previous day.

All patients must have at least one X-ray examination, with photographs being taken of the hip from different angles, and a blood test. The former provides the surgeon with an essential pre-operative guide to the actual state of the hip-joint. The latter is essential for determining the patient's blood group and Rhesus factor for any blood transfusion needed in the course of the operation. Both tests are normally carried out in the hospital booked for the operation.

Very occasionally, a surgeon, not fully satisfied by the information provided by the X-rays, will ask for a CT scan. The initials stand for computerized tomography: the process involves rotating a special X-ray unit around the body of the patient, so as to produce a succession of images which are then resolved by a computer to produce cross-sections of the hip-joint.

The process is relatively time-consuming, the apparatus is elaborate and supervision by a consultant radiologist is required. This means substantial extra costs (which will add to the bill of a private patient). In practice, conventional X-rays are normally more than adequate, but when these suggest some unusual complication, a CT scan may help considerably in planning the operation. In such a case, the scan is likely to be carried out in the hospital the day before the operation.

A patient may be asked to donate blood in advance. This will require a number of visits to a specialist blood centre, beginning several weeks before the operation. The advantage is that with any transfusion patients then receive their own blood.

Medical History

Given the age of most THR patients, their general state of health is often less than perfect. Some time before the operation, patients will be questioned about their previous medical history: this may be part of the first consultation, but if so, it is likely to be repeated at a later stage. The task is normally delegated to a junior doctor, who may spend half an hour or more asking questions relating to a patient's entire life – so it helps to have a good memory. At the same time, the family doctor can be asked for a print-out of the computer record of past treatment – this may be sent to the hospital consultant as a matter of course.

Depending on the information provided, a patient may be sent to the appropriate departments of the hospital for further tests: these can include chest X-rays, electro-cardiographs and the analysis of urine. (In many orthopaedic departments, these are routine for all THR patients at some time during the two or three months preceding the operation.) Because such a wide-ranging examination can disclose any number of conditions – high blood pressure, diabetes, chronic kidney disease – affecting vital organs, it is critically important for indicating to the anaesthetist any special precautions to be taken in the course of the operation. Occasionally the tests lead to the THR being postponed, if not cancelled, simply because the associated trauma is more than the patient's physique can safely tolerate. (There is a 35 per cent chance of death if a THR is carried out within three months of a heart attack, for example.)

Planning the Return from Hospital

In the weeks immediately before the operation, patients should begin to prepare for life at home after discharge from hospital. A critical factor here is whether there will be anyone at home to care for the patient. Ideally this will be a spouse in good health, ready to assume more than his or her fair share of domestic chores. Other members of the family, particularly grown-up children, may also be able to help. Even in such favourable cases, steps should be taken in advance of the operation to make the home suitable for a THR patient just discharged from hospital.

The main factor to take into account will then be the patient's restricted power of movement. In particular, the household should be organized so that any movement requiring a patient's torso to be bent at an angle less than 90 degrees to the leg on the operated side is avoided. In everyday life such a movement is commonplace, and is involved in such actions as putting on socks, tying up shoelaces, picking up things from the floor, getting up from a low chair or bed, getting into or out of a bath, taking a shower, or sitting on a toilet.

The way to cope is to borrow or buy special accessories, at the same time making necessary adjustments to lifestyle. There is a simple apparatus for putting on socks or stockings, and shoelaces can be avoided by wearing slip-on footwear (such as loafers) to be put on with the help of a long shoehorn. A 'helping-hand' – a sort of stick with a pincer at the far end, operated by a hand-grip – will pick up almost anything.

Desk or table chairs with arms are much better than any alternative. A low bed should be raised up by wooden blocks placed under the legs, a bathroom or shower cabin can be fitted with plastic or metal hand-holds screwed into the wall, and an adjustable plastic board can be fitted to make a firm seat resting on the sides of a bath. The level of a toilet pedestal can be raised by placing an adjustable plastic seat on top of it. It also helps to have a medical urine bottle or bed pan at the bedside for use at night.

Even with all these gizmos, it is essential to have someone around to help in the early days after discharge from hospital. For one thing, cooking and shopping will be beyond the newly returned patient for several weeks. One reason is that the patient will only be able to move around with the help of crutches (which should also be lined up before admission to hospital).

Walking with Crutches

You should learn how to walk with crutches as soon as possible. (This may also help a seriously arthritic patient with mobility problems.) The best thing to do is to ask for a lesson from a physiotherapist, thereby anticipating what you will be taught during the period of recovery in hospital.

The general principle governing the use of crutches is simple. To point out that they must be used to take the weight off the leg on the operated side may be stating the obvious, but it is still worth saying. The way to do this is to place both crutches on the ground, a step in front of the body, so that this leg can then be placed between them, leaving at the same time sufficient space for the good leg to take a full step forward. Then, with the good leg taking a step forward, to stop in a position where it can best take the whole weight of the body, the process is repeated until the patient's destination is reached. This is no more than the normal process of walking, with the two crutches moving alongside, and in phase with the leg on the operated side.

It will be seen that with this process no weight at all need be placed on the foot on the operated side. Although this is certainly required of patients recovering from a fracture (so that no stress is placed on the broken bone during the period of healing), a THR patient should begin to place some weight on the foot on the operated side as soon as possible. This will help embed the prosthesis, at the same time restoring both the thigh muscles to their normal condition, and function and mobility to the operated side of the body. All this, however, belongs to the post-operative phase, explained in Chapter 8.

Business Affairs and Current Medication

It is also a good idea for you to have your business affairs (including your will) in good order even at household level. Payment should be arranged for outstanding bills, and friends and relatives informed of the impending operation. (This also has the advantage that a surprising number will come and visit in hospital). Patients may also be able to give a telephone number where they can be reached once in hospital. (The hospital will certainly require telephone numbers for reaching the closest members of a patient's family.)

On the medical side, a patient on any form of medication should check whether this is compatible with the demands of the operation and its aftermath (which is likely to involve a number of different drugs, including, where necessary, anticoagulants).

> Hospitals commonly require a THR patient to spend the better part of the day before the operation subject to various hospital protocols involved in advance planning for surgery. Practice varies from one hospital to another: where one will submit all patients to the same procedures, without regard to their diverse medical histories, another will make every patient a separate case, so that for some the protocols will add up to very little.

Since admission means a succession of overnight stays, patients should pay special attention to packing beforehand. Several pairs of pyjamas or nightdresses, and comfortable easy-to-put-on slippers are essential, whereas a change of clothes is much less so. A sponge bag, with hairbrush and comb, toothbrush and toothpaste and shaving equipment for men, are also indispensable (check in advance that electric accessories can be kept charged). Almost any hospital now has a leaflet, which should be read with great care, telling all this to prospective patients. The leaflet should also give details of visiting hours and telephone access both to patients and those looking after them.

Almost as important for the welfare of the patient are books and other reading matter, a Walkman (with headphones) and a few favourite CDs and any other diversions to help pass the time. Remember, however, that a hospital patient has very little space to store things. Clutter must be kept to a minimum. At the same time, valuable objects, whether jewellery or credit cards, should be left at home. In a hospital, people – patients, staff, visitors or even unwelcome intruders – are coming and going all the time, and any patient is bound to keep the company of a wide selection of people, honest or dishonest, whom he or she has never met before. If, in principle, access to the wards is limited, supervision can never be 100 per cent effective. The person who steals your wedding ring could just be the patient in the next bed, or, more likely, one of his or her visitors. Even prisoners are on occasion admitted to hospital, although they are then closely watched (with normal freedom of movement restricted).

Once admitted to hospital, the patient's role is largely passive. Routine checks of temperature, pulse rate and blood pressure will start almost immediately and be repeated two or three times a day until discharge. New blood samples or X-ray photographs may be taken, enquiries will be made about diet restrictions and food preferences, and one way or another the patient will receive quite a lot of attention. Nursing staff will also be on call night and day.

Preparation for the Operation Itself

Finally, the patient must be made ready for the actual operation: no food will be allowed for at least twelve hours, and only the odd glass of water during this final period. The part of the body where the incision will be made is often shaved, and – depending on the time of the operation – sedatives may be allowed to ensure a good night's sleep. A few minutes before leaving the ward for the operating theatre, the patient must put on a special upper garment, a sort of shirt fastened round the body with Velcro. Then, with only a sheet covering the patient, the bed will be wheeled along long passages, taken into and out of lifts, to the swing doors of the operating theatre. There, the patient is handed over by the ward nurses to specially trained theatre assistants wearing their own distinctive clothing: a new world is entered within the confines of the hospital. What then happens is described in Chapter 7.

7
The Operation

As a patient suffering from arthritis of the hip, you will find a remarkable amount of literature – much in the form of pamphlets – relating to your condition. Nonetheless, the information packs provided by hospitals where THRs are regularly carried out tell you very little about the actual operation, so this is what I will cover in this chapter.

With a normal THR, the surgeon, in the space of an hour or two, achieves a radical transformation of the anatomy of the hip – as illustrated by Figure 5. This will be 100 per cent effective in eliminating the cause of your distress – although, inevitably, there is a downside, which is also described here. But then, during the critical hour or two of the operation itself, you will be powerless and, if subject to a general anaesthetic, not even conscious. The operation, by its very nature, will proceed without any form of cooperation on your part (although this may well be essential both before and after it).

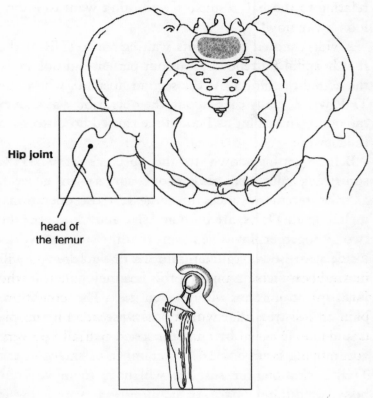

Figure 5
The structure of the pelvis and the fit of an artificial hip-joint

What interest is there, then, in knowing in any detail what the surgeon is doing at any given stage? Before going into the operating theatre, you will know that your hip-joint will be replaced by a prosthesis, an artificial device to be embedded in your body: what more do you need to know?

At this stage, I give you the standard TV warning

relating to football results, 'if you don't want to know, look away now'.

A video shown to patients waiting for a THR at the first hospital I attended as an out-patient did not show the actual operation. At the second hospital, where the THR was actually carried out, the operation was shown on video, and as far as I could see caused no distress to the viewers.

Before getting down to the specifics of a THR, something must be said about surgery in general. Despite recent advances in surgery, most operations, including all THRs, are both invasive and traumatic: the two go together. Invasive means that the surgeon works inside your body; traumatic means that in doing so he inevitably inflicts an injury – this is a major reason why your operation is not without some risk. The unbearable pain and distress that would otherwise accompany the trauma are avoided by anaesthetics, which also prevent you moving your body. (At a number of stages in the THR operation, the surgeon will have to move your body, or different parts of it, in various ways: this is often one of the assistant surgeon's tasks.)

With the steady increase in the number of THRs in the last thirty years or so, it has become a standard operation within the capability of almost any qualified orthopaedic surgeon. If you are operated on in a teaching hospital this is likely to mean that the operation itself will be carried out by a trainee surgeon, supervised by a qualified consultant. If it were otherwise, newly qualified orthopaedic surgeons would be appointed to vacancies in other hospitals, without ever having carried out a THR.

Teaching hospitals tend to be large and located in cities, where, of course, many THR patients live. In medical terms such hospitals score very highly and the consultants are the top people in the profession. This means that medical risks, in any treatment, are relatively low. As a patient you have to accept that this, when the case arises, compensates for the fact that the operation may not be carried out by a fully qualified surgeon. Nonetheless, the consultant, who is present throughout the operation, remains responsible for you. In principle you have the right to know beforehand who will do the actual operating.

The Role of the Anaesthetist

The part played by anaesthetics is so important that a specialist anaesthetist is involved in all major surgery. His task is twofold: first, by applying the appropriate means, he must ensure that you feel no pain; second, having abolished pain, he must monitor all the vital functions of your body, so that any crisis arising in the course of the operation can be dealt with.

The first can be achieved by either general or local anaesthesia. In both cases the drugs used are effective within a very short period of time and their effect – in comparison with other medications – also wears off very quickly. This is greatly to the advantage of both the patient and the surgeon.

With a general anaesthetic, the operation of your central nervous system will be reduced to a level at which you will be completely unconscious of the surgery being carried out. This result is achieved by the administration of a gas, such as Fluothane, which you will inhale throughout the operation at a rate controlled by the anaesthetist. At the same time, oxygen will be supplied directly to your lungs by a breathing tube passed through your mouth into the trachea.

General anaesthesia may reduce both blood pressure (hypotension) and heart rate (bradycardia). This should be indicated to the anaesthetist by the monitoring instruments, which function throughout the operation. With the standard apparatus at hand in the operating theatre the necessary counter-action can then be taken. For the anaesthetist this is all in the day's work and you will notice nothing. While recovering from the operation, you may suffer from nausea and vomiting, but this can be helped by appropriate medication.

Local Anaesthesia

Local anaesthesia relies on drugs injected or applied in the region to be operated upon: these suppress sensory nerve impulses, so that your brain receives no signal of the trauma inflicted by the operation. In other words you feel nothing, although you may remain conscious. Your motor nerves are suppressed at the same time, so that there is no chance of the muscles in the same region being activated.

Where local anaesthesia in used in a THR, the region subject to it comprises the entire lower half of the body. This is generally achieved by a spinal injection, using a very fine needle inserted between two of the lower vertebrae.

The actual site defines the 'block' within your body

that is subject to the effects of the anaesthetic. You will find that the effect of the anaesthesia then moves upwards through your body until this point is reached – a process taking between ten and twenty minutes according to the particular anaesthetic chosen. Plainly this upper limit to the block must be such as to ensure complete anaesthesia for the site of the operation, and as the anaesthetic begins to take effect you may be asked whether you still feel anything at different points. Only when you feel nothing at all is it safe to proceed with the operation.

After the operation the effect of the anaesthetic wears off in the reverse order, but over a rather longer period of time. You will note this when it comes to recovering sensation in your feet, and also moving them (important for discovering possible damage to the sciatic nerve).

With a local anaesthetic, a sedative such as Dormicum can be injected, so that you sleep throughout the operation. This is elective, but almost all patients make this choice. After the effect of the anaesthetic wears off, a headache, which can last as long as a week, is the most common side-effect. This occurs in fewer than 10 per cent of all cases – and medication is available to alleviate it. The fact that incidence is substantially higher for younger patients means that for the great majority of THR patients, the risk is reduced even further.

A number of advantages are claimed, perhaps questionably, for local anaesthesia: stress response and blood loss can be lower, and the same may be true with the incidence of post-operative thrombo-embolism. On the other hand, the way the anaesthesia

wears off often leads to urine retention, a problem
looked at on page 113. Backache, occasionally, is also
a problem.

As so often happens in medicine, the choice between
general and local anaesthesia is governed by a trade off
between the advantages and disadvantages of each
method. With most THRs either method is possible, but
the choice is seldom left to the patient. In the English-
speaking world general anaesthesia is probably used
with a greater proportion of patients than on the conti-
nent of Europe, but even so the present trend seems to
be towards local anaesthesia; no doubt, at international
conferences, anaesthetists argue the respective merits of
the two methods.

Whatever the usual practice in a hospital, any anaesthetist, in
special circumstances, will choose the non-standard method and
have no difficulty in applying it. This happened when Stephen
Hawking broke his hip at the beginning of 2002: general anaesthesia was impossible because in 1985, following a bout of
pneumonia, he had undergone a tracheostomy – an operation
preventing normal breathing. The operation to pin his fractured
hip could then only be performed under a local anaesthetic.

Stephen Hawking described his 'ordeal' – the word used in *The
Times* report (12 January 2002) – as 'like hearing a Black & Decker
drill', and to his personal assistant 'the operation sounded horrific
because he was conscious throughout'. I know it all because my
THR was carried out under a local anaesthetic and I did not opt
for a sedative: 'ordeal' is something of an over-statement, for you
feel absolutely nothing, and a curtain hides the whole operative
procedure. When I heard the 'Black & Decker' I was pretty
detached: I have certainly experienced worse ordeals.

If there is a British bias towards general anaesthesia, this may be because this is what patients – or more likely the surgeons – themselves prefer; my own preference (and that of my anaesthetist) was for a local anaesthetic and I have no regrets. I was warned that there could be disagreeable after-effects, but I did not suffer from them. As already noted, these can be just as serious, if not more so, with a general anaesthetic. Even so, it is worth repeating that today's state-of-the-art anaesthesia, whether local or general, has an extremely low level of risk attached to it.

Whatever choice is made, the anaesthetist will monitor the vital functions of your body throughout the operation, and where necessary take steps to correct any malfunction. Instruments will indicate your body temperature and blood pressure, and with your heart-beat displayed on a cathode-ray screen. All this will require you to be connected up before the operation starts, so that with a local anaesthetic you will see wires and tubes leading into different parts of you body. At the same time vast consoles, with dials and liquid crystal displays, provide information which, if meaningless to you, can be crucial for your anaesthetist or surgeon.

The Operation: Access and Preparation

Anaesthetics work quite quickly, so that the surgeon need wait no more than ten minutes or so before starting to operate. Once the surgeon begins his work, the opera-tion proceeds through a great number of steps, but first he must choose how to approach the focal point of the operation, which with a THR is the hip-joint. Any one surgeon will have his own preferred approach, but this may be abandoned for another in special cases, such as that of an exceptionally obese patient. This then establishes the general framework of the operation, such as the position both of the patient – who according to the approach chosen by the surgeon, may lie either on his or her back or side on the operating table – and of the surgeon in relation to the patient. At the same time, an assistant surgeon and a theatre sister will be present to help with the operation.

Although as a patient, you will hardly be conscious of what is happening, these are the steps which then follow.

After an antiseptic solution has been applied to the area chosen for the incision, you will be draped so that your whole lower body is covered with a sort of towelling (which is disposed of, as medical waste, after the operation), leaving a comparatively large area around the chosen site of the incision exposed. This in turn is generally covered with a see-through drape adhering directly to the skin. The object is to prevent bacteria on the surface of the skin gaining access to the site of the operation: this will be helped by appropriate antibiotics contained in the actual adhesive.

The first incision, which will generally be something over 10 cm long, is made through the drape and the top layer of skin, the location on the surface of the body being determined by the approach adopted by the surgeon. With the common posterior lateral approach to a THR the incision is made on the side of the body, sloping downwards from the backside at an angle of about 45 degrees.

Beneath the layer of skin, which is less than 5 mm thick, the surgeon encounters a much thicker layer of fat. This is cut through not with a knife, but with a special cutting diathermy, designed to stop bleeding from small blood vessels. A diathermy is a surgical instrument that operates by applying a small electric current directly to blood vessels. It is one type of a 'cautery', that is any instrument that destroys tissue by applying heat.

Loss of a blood is a problem that arises almost as soon as the incision is made, and this must be controlled throughout the operation. The lost blood may be replaced by a transfusion at the end of operation or, in urgent cases, in the course of it. (Many surgeons do their best to operate 'dry', in order to avoid one possible source of infection, but others take for granted the need for transfusion. In principle the body can lose at least 500 ml of blood without this need arising; normal bodily processes then make good the loss within a few hours.) In any case, the patient's blood group is known before the operation, and the transfusion apparatus will always be on stand-by.

The incision, having cut through both skin and fat, must then be opened to provide a window of access to the actual site of the operation. This involves drawing the two sides apart with an instrument known as a retractor. This is almost as important to

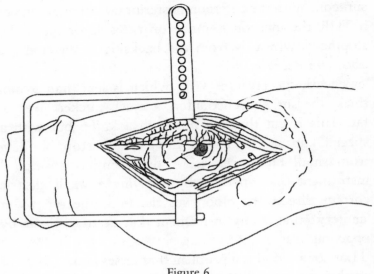

Figure 6
The Charnley Retractor

surgery as the surgeon's knife and, in the same way, comes in many different shapes and sizes. In a THR the operating site generally is kept open throughout by a fixed Charnley Retractor (illustrated in Figure 6 and named after its designer), but at certain stages additional retractors, held in place by the assistant surgeon, may be needed.

Assuming a posterior lateral approach, the next problem facing the surgeon is to find a path through the three gluteal muscles in the patient's buttocks. Given that these are responsible for movements of the thigh, they are massive and robust, although anaesthesia relaxes them to a considerable degree.

The joint, now exposed, is encased in a membrane

capsule: this must be dissected to access the actual bones comprising the hip-joint.

The femur must then be dislocated, otherwise the very close fit between the crown of the femur and the acetabulum – the part of the pelvis which it fits into – would make further progress impossible. The surgeon, helped if need be by his assistant, will achieve this result by rotating your thigh as it is pulled away, or abducted, from the mid-line of the body. (Accepting the difference in scale, this mechanical process is much the same as prising a drum-stick loose from a roast chicken – using only one's hands.) Depending upon his original approach, the surgeon will take a position either behind or in front of you; in either case he will draw the exposed crown of your femur towards him. At this stage your sciatic nerve – a major nerve of the leg – will be exposed, and the surgeon must take care not to damage it. (With some approaches the femoral nerve is more likely to be at risk, but the same principle applies.)

Your femur will then be sawn through, just below the crown, with a straight cut, using a powered saw. Because of the small space open to the surgeon, the cutting edge of the saw is very short – no more than 2.5 cm – and works by moving back and forth very rapidly.

This process will expose the medulla, or inner region of your femur (normally containing both blood and bone marrow), into which the stem of the prosthesis will be inserted. This is also the stage involving the greatest loss of blood.

The other side of the joint, where the cup of the prosthesis must be put in place, is dealt with by reaming the acetabulum, a process that includes removing arthritic cartilage and soft tissue at the centre of the cavity. The term comes from wood- and metal-working, and the process means no more than using a grinding wheel to make a circular cavity in the bone to receive the cup of the prosthesis. (Surgeons often refer to the reamer as a cheese-grater.) The actual cavity is about 50 mm in diameter.

The Prosthesis

The way is now open to implant the prosthesis, which must be described in some detail if the process is to be understood. To function as an articulated joint, the prosthesis must have two components, one for the acetabulum and the other for the femur. With most prostheses now in use, each component is modular, which means that it consists of two parts which are fitted together in the course of the operation. (Strictly, each component is a separate prosthesis, but the term is used here for the combined unit.)

The modular cup, which fits into the cavity made for it – by reaming – in the acetabulum, consists of a metal outer casing and a lining made of a special form of plastic known as HDPE (high-density polyethylene). The former is designed to fit into the acetabulum, and the latter is machined to provide a perfectly spherical concave inner surface with precisely the same dimensions as the head of the stem of the prosthesis. There must be a perfect fit between the two, otherwise the new artificial hip-joint will soon fail.

The two parts of the femoral component are the stem and the head. The stem, which is invariably metallic, is essentially a spike that will be hammered into the medulla of your femur. It has, at its exposed end, a projecting threaded boss, which screws into the head. The head, which can be either a plastic such as HDPE, or ceramic such as zirconium oxide, is perfectly spherical. The standard diameter is 28 mm, but in special cases it may be slightly larger or smaller. A threaded cavity enables the head to be screwed on to the stem, making a tight fit.

The materials used for the prosthesis must satisfy three different, if related, criteria. First, they must be chemically unreactive in the local context of the human body; otherwise contact with tissue would lead to their becoming steadily less efficient, if not outright pathogenic (causing disease). This means that only certain metal alloys, ceramics or plastics can safely be used.

Second, these materials have to be durable in the face of the stresses to which the hip is inevitably subject in everyday life. The constant friction across the two sides of the joint must not allow any sort of dust to be created. Not only would this impair the contact between the two components of the prosthesis, but there would also be the risk of secondary local inflammation. In practice there is a small post-operative risk here, and accumulated debris from a prosthesis is very occasionally a reason for a revision THR (as described on page 111).

Third, and most important, the level of friction across the artificial joint must approach, even if it cannot equal, that of a natural hip-joint. As Chapter 3 shows, the present high success rate of THRs is the direct result of John Charnley and other pioneers in the field working out how to meet all these criteria. In particular the use of low-friction polyethylene (of which HDPE is the type in current use) for the contact surfaces and acrylic cement for embedding the stem in the femur were key stages on the way to a viable operation.

Looking at these three criteria, it can be seen that the first relates to contact with bone tissue, while the second and third relate to the fit between the two components of the prosthesis. When it comes to the demands on material, these are two different cases – explaining, incidentally, the introduction of modular components consisting of two separate parts. In each case, one part, which is metallic, fits into bone tissue of the thigh or hip, which has already been prepared; only after this is done, is the part which belongs to the actual joint attached.

The extreme demands made upon a hip prosthesis define it as a high-precision product made out of specially developed materials. This explains why the present prices range from £1,500 to £3,500, a substantial part of the costs of a THR.

At the stage now reached in your operation, the surgeon will have ready for use the two separate parts of both components of the prosthesis, making four in all. The essential mechanical part of your operation can now begin, with the acetabulum, and the component of the prosthesis that fits into it, being dealt with first.

Fitting the Prosthesis

The metal outer casing of the prosthesis is first fitted into the cavity in the acetabulum made, by reaming, to receive it. Ideally it should be a tight fit, so that in most cases no cement is necessary (although in the early days of THRs, screws were used). An uncemented acetabulum component is hammered in with brute force. Where the stem component is cemented, this is known as the hybrid case, common for patients above the age of sixty-five or so.

Cement will be used for the acetabular component when the bone cannot take the strain of a tight fit, or rather the hammering required to achieve it. This is the case with patients suffering from osteoporosis, a pathological condition in which the bones are brittle and liable to fracture. (Women are particularly liable after the menopause.) To be on the safe side, many surgeons routinely opt for the use of cement for the acetabular component for almost all patients above a certain age. In such cases there is less reason for a modular component, so the surgeon may well opt for a one-piece HDPE cup.

By means of a press-fit, the plastic or ceramic lining, after being hammered in, clips securely into the metal outer casing of the acetabular component. The cup of the prosthesis will then be firmly in place and ready to receive the crown of the stem to be inserted into the femur. Nothing more needs to be done to your pelvis.

Your femur is then prepared to receive the stem of the prosthesis. This requires the removal of the tissue, mainly bone marrow, in the medulla or interior part of the bone, leaving sufficient space for the stem to be inserted. For this a special cylindrical reamer may be used.

The first insertion is provisional and is designed to find the right position for a close fit of the crown into the new artificial cup of the acetabulum. The stem is hammered in and then rotated to ensure the best angle in relation to the acetabulum. This process may be repeated two or three times before the surgeon is certain that there is an optimal fit.

A crown will then be selected, screwed on and tested for fit, and also for the optimal length of your leg once the operation is completed. For every stem there are five possible sizes of crown, according to the depth of the interior screw thread.

The provisional fitting is now over and the prosthesis is removed and temporarily set aside before permanent implanting.

Two alternative courses of action are now possible, depending upon whether or not the new prosthesis is to be cemented in position. In the early years of THR, up to the end of the 1970s, it was taken for granted that the stem should be cemented, although it was recognized that in the course of time this would make necessary a revision of the original operation – a surgical process described later in this chapter. At the same time THR was a treatment reserved for elderly patients. As Chapter 3 shows, John Charnley, who pioneered the operation in the 1960s, insisted on this – logically enough, since the condition that the operation was designed to help occurred mainly among older people.

In the course of the 1980s, with an increasing number of younger patients coming forward, orthopaedic surgeons began to consider whether the benefits of THR could be prolonged by designing a stem to be fitted so tightly into the femur that cementing could be entirely avoided. With a younger patient the natural growth of surrounding tissue could then be expected to tighten the hold on the stem of the prosthesis, or at least ensure that it did not deteriorate. The new uncemented implant promised to last a lifetime, but even if it did not and revision were to become necessary, the operation would be much simpler. Now uncemented stems are even used, occasionally, for patients over seventy-five, but as the balance of advantage here is less pronounced, many surgeons avoid this practice altogether. Others, however, work with uncemented prostheses in all but special cases, such as osteoporosis.

Most surgeons accept that the critical age for preferring an uncemented stem is about sixty-five. The trend is to accept a higher critical age, although patients as young as sixty may be given a cemented stem; this seems to be indicated for heavy smokers.

With an uncemented stem, the following steps are avoided.

A plug is inserted into the medulla at a point just beyond that reached by the lower end of the prosthesis.

This cement restrictor will prevent cement filling the whole medulla.

Adrenaline-soaked sponges are inserted to reduce blood loss. (Adrenaline, familiar as a hormone that prepares the body for 'fright, flight or fight', also has the property of constricting blood vessels and so reducing local blood supply.)

The acrylic cement used to secure the stem inside the femur is now prepared. An acrylic powder is mixed with water, perhaps with the addition of antibiotics to reduce the risk of bacterial infection.

After two minutes, the cement mix is ready for insertion into a syringe with a nozzle long enough to reach the plug. It is already becoming viscous, but it is best to deliver it before the process goes too far, so that it reaches every nook and cranny. To make this even more certain, the surgeon will apply pressure either with his finger or a rubber pestle.

The viscosity steadily increases and when, after about five minutes, the cement has the consistency of dough, the stem of the prosthesis is hammered in, taking care that it is placed at the right angle. This has already been determined by the trial fittings. Once the stem is in the right position, it must be held rigidly in place for twelve to fifteen minutes, the time needed for the cement to harden. The site is then cleaned, with the removal of the cement forced out of the medulla as the stem was hammered in.

In both cases, cemented and uncemented, the head is screwed on to the stem, which the surgeon, by an appropriate manipulation of your thigh, will fit into the cup already inserted into the acetabulum at an earlier stage. In effect, the dislocation which was necessary to access your hip for the operation is reversed.

The surgeon may insert one or more drains to remove unwanted liquid accumulating at the site of the wound. A drain consists of a small diameter (2 mm) plastic tube, led to a point outside your body, where it can discharge into a glass container. It is only needed for a few hours, and should be removed the day after the operation.

A small tube, known as a cannula, may be inserted into a vein to allow for the continuous injection of fluid during the hours following the operation. This then forms the connection for an intravenous drip with the fluid flowing under gravity from a bottle suspended above your bed.

The cannula provides the means for the blood transfusion (mentioned on page 97) made to replace the blood lost in the course of surgery. It may also be used for the first of three doses of a broad-spectrum antibiotic such as cephalosporin, used to counteract possible bacterial infection.

It only remains for the surgeon to close your wound and then apply a sterile airtight dressing to reduce any risk of infection from outside.

Birmingham Hip Resurfacing (BHR)

In the 1970s, when almost every aspect of THR was dominated by the wisdom of John Charnley, it was accepted that the operation had serious disadvantages for younger patients. The reason was simple: even the best prostheses had to be replaced after ten to twenty years, so that the prospect of revision, sometimes more than once, was a major concern.

As against this, the condition which the THR was designed to correct was mainly one that affected old people: in practice, excluding patients under sixty-five would affect only a small minority of those who suffered from arthritis of the hip. The implanting of uncemented prostheses, when it came in during the 1980s, considerably reduced the need for subsequent revision for this age group – or at least made the operation simpler if it had to be carried out. Even so, there were some who wondered whether something less radical than a THR was possible, and so alternative less radical procedures were developed and used with some success.

At the beginning of the 1990s, the challenge was taken up by two Birmingham surgeons, Derek McMinn and Ronan Treacy, both attached to the Royal Orthopaedic and Nuffield Hospitals. Birmingham is still the main centre for hip resurfacing, but BHR is now carried out by Justin Cobb, attached to London's Middlesex Hospital, and by other surgeons elsewhere – not only in the UK, but in the rest of the world. Its proponents, such as McMinn and Cobb, particularly emphasize its capacity to restore top sportsmen and women (who are particularly vulnerable to arthritis of the hip at a relatively young age) to their original level of performance. There seems hardly to be any lower age limit to the patients accepted for the operation.

In the operation itself, the approach to the hip-joint is the same as that for a THR. Then, instead of sawing off the top of the femur and inserting the stem of a prosthesis into the medulla as described above, the head of the femur is placed inside a hollow metal sphere, of which the outer surface fits perfectly into an all-metal socket fitted into the acetabulum. The two components then constitute a low-friction ball and socket joint. The choice of the metal is critical. At the present stage of research and development, a cobalt-chrome alloy has proved not only to be remarkably durable, but also capable of being machined so as to provide extremely low-friction contact surfaces of quite incredible smoothness.

At first sight it would seem that the BHR, although much simpler, lacks some obvious advantages of a conventional THR. The idea goes back at least as far back as the 1970s, but the results produced by surgeons who tried resurfacing were then unsatisfactory. The restriction to metallic materials for the two contact surfaces, and the much greater diameter of the ball and socket – up to twice that of a conventional Charnley prosthesis – could mean an unacceptably high level of friction. Cobalt-chrome has now solved the friction problem, and the much larger diameter greatly reduces the risk of dislocation in the months, if not years, following the operation. In the first ten years there has not been a single case.

Friction can be reduced still further by thick film lubrication, and with nearly 2,000 BHR operations over nine years in the 1990s, no wear has been observed on retrieved bearings, while at the same time there has been no significant increase in the patients' blood metal ion levels. The prosthesis, being both all metal and much larger, is remarkably heavy, but as a patient, you would not be aware of this.

The BHR prostheses are mainly produced by a British firm, Finsbury Orthopaedics. Mike Tuke, who set up this firm, started his professional life as a researcher in biomechanics at Imperial College, London. He is not only the CEO, but also the principal designer. His success owes much to his close collaboration with the Birmingham surgeons. The prostheses manufactured by Finsbury Orthopaedics, which extend across the whole field of joint replacement, are now used worldwide.

One still asks, is there a downside to all this? It is still too early to be sure. Since with a normal THR the need for revision hardly occurs within ten years, and the actual period may be twenty years or more, the results of a nine-year survey, which is all that time allows for with BHRs, are still problematic. They are nonetheless very encouraging, although compared to some 70,000 THRs every year, the number of BHRs is small. Their contribution to the treatment of arthritis of the hip is still somewhat marginal, but in the course of time it is certain to become less so. For the young active athletic patients who define the margin, the BHR is no doubt the optimal solution to their problem.

For most patients THR is a first-time operation. Unfortunately, a prosthesis, particularly if uncemented,

In addition, impressed by its record of success, surgeons are now beginning to carry out BHRs with older patients. Given how much longer we oldies live these days, we too are entitled to benefit from the durability of the all-metal prosthesis, to say nothing of enjoying a much lower risk of dislocation.

does not last indefinitely, so sooner or later, a new operation may be necessary. This so-called 'revision' means fitting a new prosthesis, but the operation, although basically the same, is less straightforward. For one thing, revision patients are likely to be older, with medical histories less favourable to surgery. The removal of the old prosthesis can be difficult, and there are other problems not occurring the first time round (although, on the other hand, sawing and reaming should be avoided.)

The proportion of revisions is now approaching 50 per cent. In spite of all the extra hazards there seems to be no upper age limit, and revision THRs have been performed on patients aged ninety and over.

8
After the Operation

One of your main concerns is certain to be how you will progress, in the hours, days, months and even years, following your THR operation. In principle things should only get better, but it is not quite straightforward all the way. In this game of Snakes and Ladders, there are certainly many more ladders than snakes, but the snakes are there all the same.

The First Phase: Recovery in Hospital

Your life after the operation begins in the recovery room, where you will remain until the effects of the anaesthetic have worn off – a process generally lasting an hour or two. During this time you will receive a good deal of attention. For one thing the surgeon will want to know whether the actual operation has caused a club foot. This does not happen often, but when it does, immediate remedial treatment is essential.

Possible after-effects of the anaesthetic, although much less serious in the long run, can make you quite unhappy for several days. A general anaesthetic can lead to nausea, and a local anaesthetic can leave you either with a severe headache or back pain at the site of the spinal injection. In these cases medication can reduce your misery, but time is the real cure. Fortunately most patients are spared these trials, although there will always be some level of discomfort after you are wheeled back to the ward.

At this stage, a number of tubes will lead away from different parts of your anatomy. There will be an infusion lead in one arm, enabling a constant drip feed from a bottle suspended above the bed – a scene familiar from hospital soaps on TV. At a point close to the incision (now protected by a large surgical dressing) another small plastic pipe will lead from inside your body to a small container clipped to the edge of the bed. This is the drain, designed to remove unwanted body fluids from the site of the operation. Some surgeons insert more than one drain; others avoid it entirely, seeing it as a possible source of bacterial infection.

If you were operated on under a local anaesthetic, you may have a catheter inserted, for one of the after-effects is to inhibit normal urination – known as retention. (A small echo-sounder that measures the volume of urine retained in the bladder will let the nurses on the ward know how long the catheter must remain in place.) You may be reassured to know that all this plumbing does not cause any pain; it is inconvenient rather than uncomfortable, and in any case it is not likely to be needed for longer than the first twenty-four hours after surgery. Very occasionally retention persists, sometimes – with male patients – to the point of requiring the removal of the prostate.

Once back on the ward, your well-being is likely to be affected by two rules. The first is the requirement to lie on one's back, with the legs apart; this is helped by a large triangular pillow – the so-called abduction pillow – placed between them. The second rule follows from the first; a patient, even when allowed to sit up, must not cross the leg on the operated side over the other leg.

Most surgeons regard these rules as essential for preventing any possible dislocation of the new artificial hip-joint, but when it comes to sleeping positions, you may be allowed to listen to your own body when choosing what is most comfortable. Lying on the operated side is almost always safe, since in this position the leg is kept immobile by the weight of your own body. The disadvantage is that the position is uncomfortable – so much so that you may well need a painkiller, such as paracetemol, or a sedative, before going to sleep.

The risk of dislocation, although steadily decreasing, continues into the indefinite future, but certainly after two or three months you can safely choose any sleeping position. You may even, with due care, cross the operated leg over the other one.

Normal eating and drinking is generally possible within twelve hours, and a cup of tea can be enjoyed almost immediately after you return to the ward from the recovery room. Occasionally recovering normal bowel action is a problem, which if it persists longer than a day or two may require remedial treatment. In general, however, you should be taking part in the normal hospital routine from the beginning of the day following the operation. At the same time you will be disconnected from all the plumbing, and with a new surgical dressing on the wound will be able to change into normal nightwear. Routine monitoring of blood pressure, temperature and pulse, at four-hour intervals, will probably continue until discharge from hospital.

On the first post-operative day, you will be wheeled, bed and all, to the hospital's X-ray department. The photographs taken should then confirm that the prosthesis is properly embedded – something that the surgeon will be keen to know.

Physiotherapy

The physiotherapist will also visit for the first time. At this stage you will be taught how to sit up and get out of the hospital bed. Helped by either a Zimmer frame or crutches, and the physical support of the physiotherapist, you will first stand on the floor and even walk a few uncertain steps – returning to bed with a sigh of relief.

Later in the day the physiotherapist may return to repeat the process, with a view to allowing you from the following day to make short journeys – accompanied always by a nurse – to the bathroom or toilet. On this day and those that follow it, the physiotherapist will teach you how to be more ambitious with walking, if at all possible with crutches, so that, for instance, you will learn how to go up and down stairs. At the same time the physiotherapist should begin to explain the exercises (described later in this chapter) to be carried out after returning home. These are really important for restoring function and mobility to the operated side of the body.

Post-Operative Reactions

In the days following the operation the leg may swell up; this is a normal bodily reaction, which should subside without any special treatment. If, however, the leg becomes red from inflammation, particularly in the area around the incision, this is a danger signal, indicating possible bacterial infection – with the consequences already discussed in Chapter 7.

The hospital staff will certainly be on the look-out for any DVT danger signals requiring emergency treatment. This is particularly important for patients with a history of cardiac problems, whose medication may have been interrupted over the immediate operative period.

In general, there are differing views about how seriously this risk of blood-clot formation should be taken. The use of a standard anticoagulant, such as heparin – which is administered by injection – may be judged sufficient, particularly if you are also wearing elastic stockings. The alternative is to use a drug such as coumarin, which can be taken orally. This has the advantage that the course of treatment can be continued indefinitely after you are discharged from hospital.

The problem with this approach is that to find the right dosage, the patient's blood must be continuously monitored as long as the treatment lasts. In principle, resumption of normal movement in the post-operative period should reduce the risk to a safe level, without there being any need for such prolonged treatment. This is the guiding principle, accepted by the majority of British orthopaedic surgeons and adopted by the NHS, with occasional critical cases being dealt with as they arise.

Returning Home

The immediate post-operative phase ends when you are discharged from hospital. The question is, at what stage of recovery is this possible? If you are fortunate, you may be up and about, in a limited sort of way, two days after surgery. You will be able to wear normal clothes during the daytime, sit at a table for meals, take a shower or use an invalid toilet without assistance. Needless to say, you will still be walking everywhere with crutches.

If you make good progress, you may be discharged as early as the fourth day after the operation. This will only be possible if you can move around on crutches comfortably and with a good sense of balance. You will also need to be able to get into the passenger seat of a car. (Needless to say, driving is impossible at this stage.)

Getting into a car should be done with great care. The seat should be pushed far back, the back lowered two or three notches, leaving room for comfortable positioning, without unduly bending the leg on the operated side. (Remember the critical angle of 90 degrees from Chapter 7.) The correct way is to sit first on the car seat, with the legs still outside; these can then be swung round, turning the body at the same time – clockwise in the UK – to sit comfortably in the passenger seat.

Car accessory shops sell a special cushion, which makes this process somewhat easier, and even without this it helps to have a small cushion to raise the level of the car seat.

Throughout the process, the car driver should be giving you physical support. All this will apply for some weeks after you return home, not only to you as a passenger, but also as a driver, once this is permitted (after the procedure outlined in page 124).

Living Alone

Much of what I have said above assumes that you have a home to go to where someone will be around to look after you, night and day. Unfortunately, given the age and family circumstances of many THR patients, you may not be in this position. A surgical ward can be flexible to some degree, in allowing you a longer stay in hospital, but this sort of bed-blocking seriously lowers the hospital's capacity to admit other patients.

One answer to this problem is for you to go to a special orthopaedic rehabilitation unit, with less intensive nursing, where you can stay until the point is reached that you can cope alone at home – albeit with visiting help arranged by the local council. Even so, it will be several weeks before this stage is reached. The full dimensions of this problem are discussed in Chapter 6, but now is the time to see how you can get by once you have arrived home.

The Second Phase: Rehabilitation at Home

Once you arrive home after the THR operation, you have every right to look forward to resuming normal everyday activities – most of them extremely mundane. All this takes time. There are any number of published guidelines (including on the Web) as to how many weeks should pass before one or other of these activities can be taken up again. However, as I said in the Introduction, every patient is different, so whereas you may be able to walk without crutches a fortnight after the operation, you might instead have to wait several weeks before you can do so. (This will certainly be the case if you have an uncemented prosthesis.) The same will apply to many other activities that in normal life you take for granted.

At the same time, you are likely to be concerned about the rate at which the pain and discomfort, such as follow almost any major operation, will decline. For a period of several weeks, sleep may well be a problem, particularly if you avoid lying on the non-operated side of your body. During this period, which should not last beyond the first two months after the operation, standard painkillers such as paracetamol can help considerably. Sleeping tablets, to be prescribed by your GP, can also be taken before going to bed. To reduce the risk of dependency, the course should not last longer than two months.

Most important of all, you will have to learn to use your body once again, with the new hip. This process is not as straightforward as you might think. In particular, aches and pains not experienced before the operation may arise at various stages. A pain in the small of the back is one example; getting up from a chair, or out of bed, may also lead to acute discomfort for half a minute or so. To deal with such problems, regular sessions with a physiotherapist are almost indispensable – these can be arranged before discharge from hospital. The physiotherapist, in addition to the treatment provided during the sessions, will advise not only on exercises to be carried out at home (such as those at the end of this chapter), but also on the resumption of such key activities as driving.

Although times vary from one patient to another, the order in which activities can be resumed is much the same for all patients. During the first few days at home, the patient will certainly need help in moving around, although inside the house or flat, one crutch, supporting the operated side of the body, may well be sufficient. As early as two or three weeks after your operation, even this may prove unnecessary.

For a much longer period, you must always take care about getting up from chairs (preferably with arms), into or out of bed (preferably raised on blocks), carrying heavy objects or picking things up from the floor or from floor level. Showers are better than baths and, if the shower is above the bath, then a hand-hold fixed into the wall is helpful for stepping into the bath. A special seat, which fits across the bath, can also help. Speciality shops supply all these things.

In all such activities two things must be avoided: crossing the leg on the operated side over the other one; bending the upper body forward at an angle of less than 90 degrees to the leg on the operated side. When getting up from a chair it helps to put the leg on the operated side slightly forward; this allows the other leg to take a greater share of the weight. Getting into or out of bed should always be on the operated side of your body.

To get into bed, first sit on it and then swivel the legs round, leading with the non-operated side; to get out, reverse the process, this time leading with the operated side, but in standing up, putting more weight on the non-operated side. (These movements follow the same principle for getting into and out of cars.) In the first weeks at home, patients should be supported by at least one crutch, or the arm of someone else at home.

Given all these considerations, you will find that living at home again requires a certain adjustment from your old lifestyle. Putting on socks is a problem, but it can be solved with a simple apparatus available from medical supply stores. For shoes, choose loafers rather than lace-ups and use a shoehorn. At home, also, take particular care with thresholds and slippery mats: a fall can mean dislocation. If something is dropped on the floor, either use a helping-hand (as described in Chapter 6) or ask someone else to pick it up. The same is true of taking things from the lowest shelves in supermarkets. In such a case do not be ashamed to ask for help, even from people you do not know: just say first, 'I am just getting over a hip operation', and the help, in 99 cases out of 100, will be willingly given. At home, someone else should get things out of the oven, the bottom of the refrigerator, or the lowest shelf of a cupboard or bookcase. (Of course, if any of these are at eye level, there is no problem.)

Extra Support

Once at home you may be entitled to support from home helpers and carers. This will come either from your local council or from an outside agency, but in either case you will be billed by the council. To meet the cost there is a care allowance of up to about £50, no matter what your income, and you can use this also on help arranged for privately. The recognized council rate for domestic services is about £10 per hour, so the care allowance will not go all that far. If more help is needed and you cannot afford it, you will have to make a special application for support from the council.

Getting Around Outside the Home

Walking is definitely to be recommended, because of the need to exercise your new hip-joint. As the weeks go by, distances will become longer, but within two or three months, a mile or two should certainly be possible. To avoid dislocation, take extra care not to trip or stumble. Once again, every patient is different, so trust your own judgement and listen to your own body. Steps, particularly on the operated side, should be as long as possible, and the body should remain upright. Going up and down stairs is also good exercise, but remember the 90 degree rule.

Travelling over longer distances is more of a problem. The simplest way is to be a passenger in a car, getting in and out in the way explained on page 118. Driving again after a THR is another question, dealt with below. Public transport, particularly on buses, is definitely hazardous, and the rush hour, with standing passengers, is best avoided for as long as possible: the same goes for cycling. Trains are easier, particularly when the platform is at the right level, with not too wide a gap separating it from the train. With the tube and other local or suburban services, getting off at the right station requires a lot of care, particularly when the train is crowded. Escalators are also a problem, especially when going down, where there is a risk of losing one's balance. Lifts are generally easier, but avoid getting caught as the doors close (even though they should then open again automatically).

For THR patients, flying is probably the easiest form of public transport; passengers are guaranteed a seat, and the aeroplane does not take off until all are seated and belted in. At the same time, airline personnel can offer special help (which is best asked for at the check-in). Above all, be patient – don't worry about being the last off the aeroplane. Remember that when travelling away from home a suitcase on wheels is almost indispensable (but remember always to ask for help when it must be lifted – say from an airport carousel).

Taking up driving again after a THR requires the permission of the Drivers Medical Unit of the DVLA at Swansea. As soon as possible after the operation, you should notify the Unit (telephone 08702 400009 or postal address, Swansea SA99 1TU) and ask for a medical questionnaire. This must be completed either by the orthopaedic surgeon or your family doctor, and sent back to the unit once you have been judged as fit to drive again. According to the answers given, a decision will be taken and you will be notified. The procedure is not unduly protracted, but a new medical driving licence may be required. With a favourable wind you may even be driving again within three weeks of the operation, but you will probably have to wait somewhat longer.

Sex Life after a THR

To begin with, the aftermath of the operation will leave you with little sexual desire; this is unlikely to come back until several days after discharge from hospital. At the same time, given your age, sexual activity may already be at a relatively low level, if it has not been given up altogether. Having said all this, sexual capacity and arthritis of the hip are not physiologically related, so difficulties in resuming sex after a THR are likely to be largely psychological – although not any less real for that. This is particularly true in the long term. Nonetheless, sex is a physical activity, and one which can be particularly demanding on certain parts of the body such as your hips – and this is what counts in the short term.

If you are able to resume sex, you should certainly make clear where and how discomfort arises and expect your partner to adjust accordingly. To begin with it may be best not to have full intercourse – just see what is possible with intimate contact, and go on from there. If all other everyday activities have been resumed, say after three months, normal sex should be part of them, but here, above all, the decision is yours.

Physiotherapy and Exercise

Once you return home after being discharged from hospital you will still require physiotherapy. For this you may return to the hospital as an out-patient, or attend a local physiotherapy practice. In either case, the early sessions will be largely devoted to manipulative treatment, designed to ensure the restoration of mobility and function to your new hip-joint. Gradually the exercise bicycle and the walking platform will be introduced, and you will be encouraged to cycle and walk at a steadily increasing rate. Under the supervision of the physiotherapist, you will learn to keep your torso upright rather than leaning forward with the movement of your legs. (At this stage it helps to have been drilled by a sergeant-major in the armed forces – given their age, a common experience in the distant National Service past of male THR patients.)

More important than the physiotherapy itself (which may only add up to an hour a week) are the exercises you learn in the course of it. To enjoy the full benefit, you should allow at least half an hour a day to perform them.

Exercises

Although there are a number of different exercises, they are all designed to restore mobility and function on the operated side of your body to the level you enjoyed before you began to suffer from arthritis. This may prove to be a counsel of perfection, but following your THR you should still aim to reach a much improved level. There should be no pain either during the exercises, nor immediately following them; just listen to your own body to see how far you can go.

Now look at the actual exercises, which are a selection from those in any physiotherapist's repertoire. As shown in Figures 7a to 7h, the leg on the operated side is shaded. You should repeat each of these exercises ten times, twice every day; this may prove to be somewhat of a bind, but the effort will certainly be rewarded.

GROUP A: LYING DOWN EXERCISES

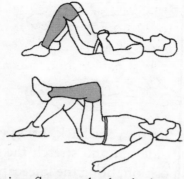

Figure 7a. Lying flat on the back, bring your knees up, keeping the soles of your feet on the floor. Then raise the leg on the operated side, keeping the knee bent at 90 degrees, remembering that the angle between the thigh and the torso should *never* exceed 90 degrees.

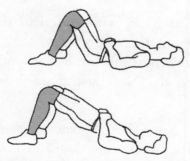

Figure 7b. Start in the same position as in Figure 7a, but raise your torso so that your body is supported by your feet and your shoulders, with the buttocks off the ground.

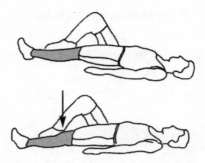

Figure 7c. Lying flat on your back, bring your knee on the non-operated side up, and stretch the operated leg right out: in this position, bring the kneecap down as far as possible.

Lying flat on your back, and starting with your legs together, move the operated leg out sideways as far it will go, with the toes pointing to the ceiling. (Not illustrated.)

Lying flat on your back, with your legs together and straight out, tighten the buttocks so that they pinch together. Hold this position for five seconds and then relax for five seconds. (Not illustrated.)

GROUP B: SITTING EXERCISES

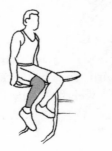
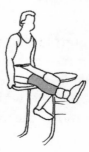

Figure 7d. Sitting on the edge of a table, with your back upright, stretch out the operated leg so that it is straight at the knee. Hold the position for five seconds.

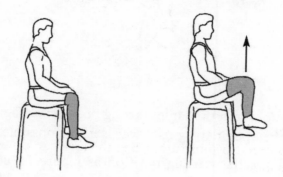

Figure 7e. Starting in the same position as Figure 7d, raise up the knee of the operated leg, but not so that the angle between your thigh and torso becomes less than 90 degrees.

GROUP C: STANDING EXERCISES

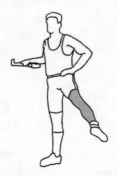

Figure 7f. Starting with your weight placed evenly on both legs, move the operated leg sideways as far as possible.

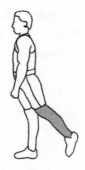

Figure 7g. From the same starting position as Figures 7f, move the operated leg backwards as far possible.

From the same starting position as Figure 7f, combine the above two exercises, by moving the operated leg first sideways as in Figure 7f, then backwards from the new position, then inwards to the position reached with Figure 7g, so that the point of your toe touches the four corners of a square. (Not illustrated.)

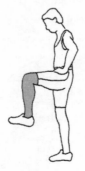

Figure 7h. From the same starting position as Figure 7f, raise upwards the knee of the operated leg.

These standing-up exercises are the most important. An upright posture must be maintained throughout, so the movement of your leg must not be allowed to carry your whole upper body with it. Since this can happen only too easily, it is a good idea to carry out standing exercises in front of a full-length mirror, wearing as few (preferably tight-fitting) clothes as possible. At least to begin with, the support of an upright chair, placed with its seat forwards, is to be recommended to help with balance. In the course of time, helped by the balancing exercises, you should dispense with the chair. It also helps greatly if the exercises are first carried out under the supervision of a physiotherapist, who will call your attention to any incorrect posture or movement.

GROUP D: BALANCING EXERCISES (TO BE CARRIED OUT WITH BOTH LEGS)

From the same starting position as Figure 7f, take a long step sideways with one leg, then bring the other leg up next to it, without placing the foot on the ground. Hold this position (standing on one leg) for five seconds. Then move the raised leg back to its original position. Repeat, reversing the roles of the two legs. (Not illustrated.)

From the same starting position as Figure 7f, raise one knee up and then stretch out the leg forwards. Move the same outstretched leg backwards as far as it will go. Bring it back to its original position, without the foot having touched the ground at any stage. Repeat with the other leg. (Not illustrated.)

The Limits to Recovery

You will naturally want to know how far the process of recovery will take you. Before the operation, you will have had to live with varying degrees of pain and discomfort, accompanied by loss of mobility and function. Your distress may have lasted for a period measured in years rather than months.

The process of rehabilitation is most rapid in the days immediately following the operation. Although you will suffer pain and discomfort for some weeks, so that sleep will not be all that easy, from the very first day your hip-joint will be completely free of arthritis – you will notice this immediately.

Long-term Prospects

Three months after your THR, when you are free from the post-operative discipline, with its restrictions on sleeping position and limb movement, you may still wonder about the degree to which your physical powers will be restored. When, if ever, will it be possible to take up old sports – golf, tennis, skiing, to say nothing of dancing?

The lesson for all THR patients is quite simple: 'don't give up' – but 'don't be too impatient either'. A balance must be struck between sloth and over-exertion. You do best to avoid comparing yourself to other patients: most of us never came near to being top mountaineers or dancers. On the other hand, do not shrink from normal outside activities, such as walking to the shops or travel-

THR may be a standard operation, but its power to restore patients' capacity for sport and physical exercise cannot be precisely defined. Partly this is a question of the patient's own will. The Earl of Limerick, who died in 2003, climbed the Matterhorn two years after his first THR and, following his second some years later, abseiled down the face of the 625 ft Canary Wharf. Just as impressively, in 2002 the 75-year-old dancer and choreographer Gillian Lynne returned to the West End stage with *Chitty Chitty Bang Bang* after not one, but two THRs. Although both were carried out by Sarah Muirhead-Allwood, a world leader in hip surgery, she would probably be quite modest in claiming credit for her distinguished patient's successful return to professional life. This was much more a triumph of Gillian Lynne's own will-power.

ling by public transport – and cycling if that was part of your life before your THR. Unless the weather is appalling, get out for at least half an hour every day, taking care not to stumble or slip. A positive attitude is the key to a good recovery. Couch potatoes, be warned!

9
The Social Dimension

As a THR patient you probably grew up with the idea
that a hospital was a residential institution where sick
people were accommodated in wards for such time –
measured in days, if not weeks – as was necessary for
their recovery from whatever condition had brought
them there in the first place. The focus was as much on
the therapeutic value of nursing, over a relatively long
period of time, as it was on the specialist treatment,
including surgery, provided by consultants. In the early
1970s John Charnley's THR patients stayed in hospital
for five weeks after the operation; today, it is more likely
to be five days.

The focus of today's medicine is on treatment, which
may be radical and invasive, such as the surgery
required for your THR. Following surgery, you should
remain in hospital only for as long as is necessary to take
care of any possible crisis, requiring more or less
intensive care, during the period of recovery from the

operation. In some fields, such as eye surgery, this is often no more than a matter of hours, with patients discharged on the day of the operation. There are now specialist eye hospitals with no beds at all for in-patients.

The emphasis then, is on discharge from hospital in the shortest possible time. Lying in bed is seen as a hindrance rather than a help. Mobility is the key to recovery, so that as a THR patient, within two days of the operation you will find yourself having a shower, using the toilet, sitting at a table for meals and getting dressed immediately after breakfast. In all this you will need help not only from nurses on the ward but also from a physiotherapist, particularly when it comes to walking with crutches.

Although by this stage you are almost ready for discharge from hospital, at least according to today's standards, you are not in any state to return home unaccompanied, let alone look after yourself without help once you get there.

After discharge from hospital the ideal scenario for you as a patient is a home with easy access from the street, with no difficult stairs to climb, and an attentive and healthy spouse or grown-up child to look after the housekeeping.

It helps also to have a family car, not only to fetch you from the hospital, but also to provide regular chauffeur service if only for your visits to the physiotherapist.

This was the scenario which, about three weeks before my own THR, I saw portrayed in a short video. The main character was a female patient, shown both pre- and post-op, about seventy years old, whose arthritic hip meant that she could no longer enjoy working in her garden. The setting presented to viewers was so opulent that one could easily imagine the BMW parked in the drive. The lady would almost certainly have opted for treatment in a private hospital outside the NHS. There, after a few days in her own room, recovering from the operation, she would have been discharged, to be driven home by her husband or some other member of her family.

On the other side of the social divide, we find a much older patient, perhaps eighty-five years old, living alone in a council flat, four floors up without a lift. No family, friends or neighbours are around to help after the THR. Returning home within a week of the operation is out of the question (even with the help of an NHS ambulance for walking patients). A day or two longer in hospital may be permitted, but the care that such a patient needs is measured in weeks rather than days.

Residential care – say in a convalescent home – is an area in which the NHS, or private insurers, are reluctant to accept responsibility. There may be public funds available in some cases, but they are not to be counted on. Otherwise patients, or their families, are left to the foot the bill, which may easily run into four figures.

All this makes it in your interest to return home as soon as possible. Regular visits by the district nurse, perhaps the physiotherapist, domestic help provided by the local council, meals-on-wheels and many other services can help make this a realistic option. A good GP's surgery should be able to provide the right contact details before you are admitted to hospital for the operation, and in any case a medical social worker, attached to the hospital, should help in lining up all these services before you are discharged.

Even so, if you are elderly and in relatively poor health, it will be some weeks after your THR before you can go out shopping or even for a walk round the block. Voluntary workers may be able to help you, but the position is still far from satisfactory. If nothing can be worked out, you may find yourself joining the vast regiment of bed-blockers who are the bane of NHS hospital administrators.

This is the hidden dimension of THR, as it is of many other conditions requiring major surgery, particularly if you are old and live alone. The government may well keep its promise to reduce waiting times to under six months, but then with the inevitable increase in the number of operations the after-care problem can only be exacerbated.

There are ways of solving this problem – many of them quite obvious – but they all cost money, and the government's health budget is already stretched to the limit of what politicians can ask taxpayers to pay for. In this situation, there will be both winners and losers. As the British population becomes steadily older, this crucial aspect of THR threatens to become ever more critical, with too few winners and too many losers. John Charnley, and those who followed him, have only solved half the problem.

The scenario is well documented: in the last twenty years or so, there has been almost a 50 per cent decline in elderly patients in NHS hospitals. Over the same period, the number in private health care institutions has increased by a factor of more than six, so that whereas this category numbered substantially fewer patients in 1980, it numbered nearly three times as many in 2000. In the same twenty years there was a comparable increase in the number of those in private or voluntary residential homes, so that these last two categories now house some 400,000 people. A very considerable number of them will have had a THR, but even after recovery they have no better place to live.

10
Private Treatment

The Consultant and the Patient

From the very beginnings of the NHS, in 1948, the medical profession, or at least its more successful practitioners, have held successive governments to ransom when it comes down to preserving the right to private practice. In more than fifty years, the position has hardly changed. With the reorganization of the NHS, presented to Parliament in the summer of 2002, the government, in spite of offering much increased remuneration to consultants, was still forced to accept almost all the terms they dictated when it came to the right to private practice.

In 2002, the spokesman for the British Medical Association was satisfied that the compromise reached between consultants and the NHS imposed no restriction on private practice, not even during a specialist's first seven years in practice, as the government had wanted. The minister had to be content with the fact that 'for the first time it is explicitly part of the contract that NHS patients come first and the NHS always has first call on a consultant's time'. However, it is not for nothing that the new restrictions have been described as 'golden handcuffs'. Only time will tell what this adds up to.

When it comes to health care in the UK, there are two different camps, that of the NHS and that of private practice. This fact tells you nothing new. However, the implications for THR need to be worked out in some detail. Although both patients and consultants can have a foot in both camps, the strategies open to them when it comes to making a choice are hardly compatible. When you choose between NHS and private treatment, you are making a one-off decision, relating to a single condition – say, arthritis of the hip. Surgeons, in dividing their time between the two camps, define a strategy that will govern their professional lives – subject always to their commitments on one side of the line or the other.

The Specialist and the Hospital

When it is a question of any major operation that requires admission to a hospital surgical ward, you are confronted with two different categories of medical treatment: the first is the operation, and the second is the nursing care you will enjoy during your stay in hospital. The two sides are obviously complementary, and the fact that the hospital also provides the operating theatre, together with supporting nursing and para-medic staff, means that during the operation you will be involved with both aspects of treatment.

Nevertheless, when it comes to private care, patients – at least in principle – must deal with the two aspects separately. First, there must be a hospital that can offer the required services, both during surgery and in the ward, at a time acceptable to the individual patient. Second, there must be surgeons, with supporting anaes-thetists, who can fit in with the hospital's timetable. As a patient you will have to negotiate separately with both sides, each with its own scale of charges and its own timetables (although there will certainly be some liaison between the two).

The surgeon, or rather his or her practice manager, should quote a fee for the operation at your very first consultation. There will be three components: first, the consultation, second, the surgery; and third, the remuneration of the anaesthetist. The three, taken together, will add up to something over £2,000, but much the greater part of this will be for the operation. There will then be another £1500, or more, for the prosthesis. The bill, adding up to some £4,000, will be sent to the patient at about the time of discharge from hospital.

During the operation your consultant surgeon will be assisted by another, who may be his registrar. The assis-tant surgeon will share the fee you agreed with the consultant, but this is a matter for the two of them to arrange between themselves. It is as well to bear all this in mind when you consider the level of the fee set by the consultant.

Although the charges made by a hospital for private treatment (which may well be the only category of treatment provided) are almost invariably stated in a booklet sent to all prospective patients, they will in practice be open-ended. In other words, in addition to the daily room charge (say £400) and that for the operating theatre (say, £500), you will be charged both for pre- and post-operative care and for drugs, dressings and all other disposable items used during and after your operation.

The total room charge will depend on the length of stay, which with a THR can be anything from six days upwards – although a stay of longer than two weeks is unusual, unless there are complications of the kind dealt with in Chapter 7.

Open-ended Charges in Private Hospitals

The uncertain factor, here, is the aggregate charge for pre- and post-operative care and for drugs, dressings and all other disposable items used during and after the operation. In fact, although with a THR there is in most cases no need for pre-operative care, at least one London private hospital requires a provisional pre-payment of £500 for this, without specifying what the treatment consists of. (Treatment, if any is needed, will of course vary from one patient to another.)

Hospitals make a similar charge for post-operative

care, by implication falling outside the scope of routine nursing. Few details are given in advance, but from my research it has become clear that the charges made by different hospitals are broadly similar in private health care.

When it comes to drugs, dressings and all other disposable items, the charge made will be around £1,000. Given that the gowns, masks, caps and gloves worn by the surgeon, the anaesthetist and the theatre nurses are all throw-away items, as are the syringes, swabs, etc., such a cost seems on the face of it quite reasonable. Yet these items cost very little – the price of a throw-away surgical gown is about £3 – and even a profligate theatre team would find it difficult to run costs up to £100, let alone £1,000.

If you are contemplating a THR outside the NHS, you may well be wondering why you are being asked to pay some £2,000, when in many, if not a majority of cases, a tenth of this amount would cover the actual costs incurred by the hospital. In practice, a private hospital reckons in advance the cost of the most expensive potential care, within the parameters of the relevant operation, say a THR. You will then be required to pay this sum as a deposit before admission. This can mean a bill in the order of £5,000. Then, after discharge from hospital, you should receive a refund for any actual shortfall in costs. This should be substantial, but whether it will be depends on the policy and practice of the hospital in question. My advice is to look into this with considerable care before you make any definite commitment.

A word of warning: all the sums quoted above are not only likely to increase over time, but also vary from one hospital to another. Do not be surprised, after paying for your THR in a private hospital, if you meet other people who paid substantially more or less than you did.

A few further facts should help. There are over 200 private hospitals in the UK in which THRs are carried out. Almost any such hospital will, if asked, supply a list of orthopaedic surgeons who regularly operate there. Any surgeon with a private practice will operate regularly in only a small number – perhaps only one – of such hospitals. The actual number will be determined largely by how many are conveniently located for the surgeon's practice; for a Harley Street consultant, for example, the number may be relatively large, given how many private hospitals there are in central London.

Which Hospital?

Although there appears to be no directory covering all private hospitals in the UK, your GP should be able to advise you about those reasonably close to your home. At the same time, a substantial number of private hospitals belong to groups such as the Nuffield Trust and BUPA, each with nearly forty hospitals.

The *Sunday Times* published a 'Good Hospital Guide' on 6 April 2003. This lists some 150 private hospitals, and for most of them states the average overall cost of a THR. The range is from just over £6,000 at the Sandringham

Hospital, King's Lynn, to just under £14,000 at the Harley Street Clinic. Even in the London area there are hospitals, such as St Anthony's, Sutton (which has a first-class orthopaedic unit), charging at the lower end of the scale.

Nuffield and BUPA have lists of all the hospitals available, and these can be consulted on the Internet. The same is true of many of the hospitals listed in the *Sunday Times* guide. What is more, each individual hospital in the Nuffield group will quote a standard charge for a THR, valid for three months. In addition, Nuffield has a financial arrangement with Barclay's Bank, allowing for the cost of the operation to be spread over a period of several years. Although you may naturally prefer a local hospital, it is worth shopping around, given how much the costs of a THR can vary from one hospital to another, even within the same group.

Prothesis Costs

The total price you end up paying may be doubled when the price of the prothesis is taken into account.

As for pre- and post-operative care, there are also considerable variations in the price of a prosthesis. The present range is from about £1,500 to £3,500. Although your surgeon may insist on his or her own choice, the trend is towards allowing you the patient a say in this matter. Although the range of prostheses available is considerable, you can learn much about their respective prices and the merits claimed for them by surfing the Web. Talk to your surgeon about this at your first consultation.

A complete THR will therefore cost a private patient somewhere between £6,000 and £12,000, and even these prices are based on very rough estimates. This compares with the sum of £4,000 or so that a hip replacement costs the NHS. In other words what you will pay for a private THR can easily be three times as much as the budgeted cost of the operation under the NHS. It is as well to look at why this is so, before considering whether, and if so how, you can beat the market in private treatment.

Once again, the same two aspects of treatment need to be considered, now reflected in the fee paid to the surgeon and the total charges made by the hospital. When talking about money – as we are now – there is no essential relationship between the two.

The Surgeon's Remuneration

Let us look first at your surgeon's fee, and – to make things simple – assume that his or her private practice consists solely of THRs. (There are one or two consultant orthopaedic surgeons who do nothing but hip operations, although some of these will be for fractures and other traumas rather than THRs.) In private practice, your surgeon will probably be content with three THRs performed in one day, so that the money earned at the end of the day will be around £5,000 – particularly if the odd consultation is fitted in as well. Out of this sum, about £1,000 will be paid to the assistant surgeon, leaving, say, £4,000, for your consultant.

Taking a 44-week working year (about standard for medical consultants) and a surgeon devoting one day a week to private practice, this will add up to well over £150,000. In terms of the money earned for any one type of treatment, such as a THR, a private practice on the side provides a full-time NHS consultant with overtime paid at many times the NHS rate. Is it any wonder that consultants fight so hard to retain their rights – and have done so from the very beginnings of the NHS?

What is more, even if one day a week of private practice is the limit agreed for new consultants, there are still established consultants who give less than half their time to their NHS commitments. This allows for annual earnings above the half a million pounds mark (in addition to remuneration for work done as a NHS consultant). There are costs attached, such as the rent of a consulting room and the salary of a practice manager, but even so, the top consultants in orthopedic surgery are very fat cats indeed; however, as they would be the first to point out, no fatter than top lawyers and accountants.

The private practice of an orthopaedic surgeon may well include trauma patients besides those accepted for elective surgery, such as a THR. Injuries in top level professional sport can demand a great deal of a consultant's time; when David Beckham needed urgent treatment for his injured foot, to be ready for the opening of the World Cup in 2002, he did not find it under the NHS (although the consultants who looked after him almost certainly had at least a part-time NHS practice). Later in 2002 Beckham's then club, Manchester United, paid £30 million for Rio Ferdinand; going further afield Real Madrid paid £36 million for Luis Figo and £42 million for Zinedine Zidane. With this sort of money at stake, every day counts and the odd £10,000 for orthopaedic surgery is peanuts!

The Bottom Line

In any event, when you are faced with consultant's bills of the order of £2,000, you must realize that this is no more than a fraction of the total charges you will be liable for once the cost of the prosthesis and hospitalization are included. If you are considering private treatment you must be prepared to pay up to £12,000, if not more, for your THR. This is about the cost of a new car, or half the annual fees at an independent boarding school – not much consolation, of course, if you never could afford life on this scale.

Two questions now require to be answered. The first is, is it all worthwhile? The second is, can anything be done to bring the costs down, once the choice is made for private treatment?

Basically what you get for your money is a surgeon of your own choice, combined with a considerable gain in time and comfort. Once you make the decision, your operation may well be performed within a month, and almost certainly with three months. Once in hospital, you will enjoy a private room, with the sort of amenities – TV, telephone, refrigerator – standard in a modern hotel. There will be few restrictions on visitors. Still, it is the time factor that is decisive: waiting a month or two, instead of a year or more, counts for much for you, the afflicted patient.

On the other hand, the operation itself will be no different from one carried out by the same surgeon in his or her NHS practice. When it comes to post-operative care, a large modern NHS hospital may in fact score higher than a private hospital, particularly in a crisis situation.

When a crisis arises it is not all that uncommon for private patients to be transferred to a large NHS hospital. The resources available, particularly when intensive care is needed, are likely to be much greater.

Now, under the new regime for NHS patients, up to 150,000 operations a year may be contracted out (at government expense) to private hospitals; these are certain to include a number of THRs. All in all, when it is a matter of clinical standards, there is little to choose between the two when it comes to a straightforward THR.

Your main advantage as a private patient is near complete freedom of choice for both surgeon and hospital. As already noted, there are some obvious limitations: a surgeon will be reluctant to operate too far from his own consulting rooms. In practice a private hospital will have a list of orthopaedic surgeons commonly making use of its facilities, and this can be very helpful to prospective patients such as yourself. I would recommend choosing a hospital first, largely on the basis of cost, convenience and the experience of family or friends.

In some cases, special rates may apply: to give one example, officers from the armed services, in service or retired, and their families, enjoy very low rates for patient accommodation at King Edward VII's Hospital in London (where the late Queen Mother had her THR at the age of ninety-seven). Such an advantage does not extend to other costs, however, and may be forfeited, in whole or in part, when the patient's costs are paid under an insurance policy – a possibility I consider in the following section.

Having found a hospital (or the private wing of an NHS hospital), you can then go on to find a surgeon, preferably one on the list of your chosen hospital. Here time can be a critical factor: a surgeon can have a long waiting list even with his private patients, whereas private hospitals – except at very short notice – can generally accommodate any time that suits a particular surgeon. All this can be discussed with your surgeon's practice manager, who can also be asked about the charges for the consultation, operation, anaesthesia and prosthesis.

At the end of the process you will have lined up a hospital and a surgeon, with an appointed day for the operation (which to begin with may be provisional) and some idea of the expected costs. The reason for uncertainty here is that neither the exact length of stay in hospital, nor the amount of additional charges, can be known in advance. (Note once again the fixed price THR offered by hospitals in the Nuffield group.)

At this stage, looking at the bottom line, you will see that almost everything is a question of time and money. If you are relatively affluent, you will have little difficulty in opting for private treatment, while, if your means are too modest, you will realize that there is no way of meeting the costs. Nevertheless, you could find yourself being able to afford private treatment by adopting a more or less radical financial strategy, say by taking out a new mortgage on your house. The Nuffield arrangement with Barclay's Bank provides another example. The question you have to answer is whether the substantially improved quality of life, during the months of waiting saved by opting for a THR in a private hospital, is worth the required financial sacrifice. A bank manager, or other financial adviser, can explain the economic implications, but at the end of the day the choice lies with you and your family.

In the particular case of THR, the majority of British patients will benefit from exemption from National Insurance (NI) contributions on account of their age. In contrast to other EU countries, this is the position of all UK residents over the age of sixty-five. The advantage is considerable. From, and including, the tax year ending 5 April 2003, for married persons in the age range sixty-five to seventy-four, the amount payable in annual tax and NI on an income of £30,000 is £5,143: under the age of sixty-five the figure would be £7,893. The difference amounts to an annual saving of £2,710: in three years this could pay for your THR as a private patient. The advantage for patients over seventy-five could be even greater. (All these figures, of course, are likely to increase over time.)

The position, needless to say, is not quite so simple. To begin with, I accept that most people in the UK never attain an income of £30,000 per annum, in which case private health care will hardly ever be an option. On the other hand, in the business and professional classes a pension at this level is common enough. What is more, although a pension generally means a loss of income, you are very likely compensated by having paid off your mortgage and no longer bearing the costs of your children's upbringing. You can also economize by moving into a smaller home. Advertisers know well that you belong to a population category with money to spend – just look at how popular cruises are as a holiday choice among older people.

There is also a demographic dimension. Rich people live longer. According to a recent survey, current average life expectancy in the Chilterns is seventy-eight where in central Glasgow it is sixty-eight. (The Chilterns area, defined by Berkshire, Buckinghamshire and Oxfordshire, also has the lowest rate of unemployment in the UK.) For every 1,000 people, this could mean ten times as many THR patients and probably ten times as many people with incomes above £30,000. The multiplier would be much greater when it comes to the number of THR patients who go for private treatment: in this part of England, the figure could be as high as 50 per cent.

If, then, you can afford private treatment, the best advice I can give you is to shop around and ask a lot of questions. Private health care is part of the market economy, which determines such matters as the occupation rate of hospital wards (much lower than under the NHS) and the fees charged by specialists. There is no reason why you should not approach private treatment in the same way as you would plan a vacation – looking at all the glossy brochures, working out possible dates and weighing up costs.

It is not much help to take a stand on principle: you may think it a scandal to pay a fee of £2,000 to a specialist whose annual income is ten times anything you ever earned, but that is the way things are in the market – and the same could be true if you ever needed a lawyer. If you are patient, you can always revert to the planned economy of the NHS (which in the long term could well be in your best interests). Some things, such as THR prostheses, cost much the same either way (although here the NHS may have some advantage from bulk contracts with suppliers). I find it astonishing that something so simple costs so much, but here we are forced to trust the manufacturers – however reluctant they appear to be to compete on price. John Charnley's first prostheses cost about £15, but this was before the inflation of the 1970s. Even so, today's prices, which start at somewhere around £1,500, do seem somewhat excessive.

Medical Insurance

A very substantial proportion – around 90 per cent – of the THRs performed outside the NHS are covered by medical insurance. The total number of such operations in any one year may be as high as 20,000. The largest of the private medical insurers, such as BUPA, have their own fact sheet on THR. For BUPA, this can be down-loaded or printed from the website, www.bupa.co.uk. (This is the source of the illustration on page 89.) Many large general insurers, such as Norwich Union, also offer a variety of medical policies. Indeed, more than 400 British insurance companies offer some medical cover. The Association of British Insurers has published its own guide on this subject, *Are You Buying Private Medical Insurance?* This can also be found on the Web, as can details of the policies offered by many insurers.

It is common practice for an employer to offer group health insurance to employees, with terms considerably more advantageous than they would enjoy if they were insured as individuals. For potential THR patients it is essential that these continue to be valid after retirement.

A word of warning: before you look at possible insurance cover, you must be absolutely clear on one point. No policy will cover a pre-existing condition and, what is more, you must reveal any such condition on the proposal form. This puts paid to any idea of your taking out cover for a THR *after* the first symptoms of arthritis of the hip have appeared. In any case, if you want to take out new medical insurance, the insurance company is almost certain to require a medical examination.

The exclusion clause may be drastic in its effects, even when the policy is taken out years before the condition requiring a THR first appears. To give one example, if as a child you suffered from Perthes' disease (which leads to deformity of the crown of the femur), you may be excluded from cover, even if in later life you appear to have made a complete recovery. Quite simply, the risk of arthritis of the hip in Perthes cases is too high to be acceptable to most insurers.

One reason why the NHS finds it so difficult to cover costs is that it accepts *all* risks, something that no insurance company can afford to do.

A further hazard, particularly for older patients, is that the risks covered may increase very substantially with age. This is certainly the case with THRs. An insurer writing a policy for the thirty to forty age group will hardly be worried about THR; for the seventy to eighty age group this will be a major part of the risk covered, particularly for women. Given the costs of the operation, this is a major reason for the much increased premiums charged to this category. This is true even with policies that have been running for years. For example, if you took out a policy at the age of twenty you may expect to see premiums increase by a factor of five by the time you reach eighty – and that is without allowing for inflation. To begin with the annual rate of increase will be quite low, but it will begin to rise sharply around retirement age. In hard cash this means that top cover can easily cost seventy- to eighty-year-olds more than £2,000 a year. Even the cheapest cover will be around £1,500, whereas twenty- to thirty-year-olds (who seldom need THRs) will pay about a fifth of this. Of course the insurance will cover much else besides THRs, but it is worth noting that it will never cover chronic conditions.

The problem is that the contract runs for only one year. There will almost certainly be a renewal clause, but the rights guaranteed to the insured are unlikely to extend for more than ten years. Taking the greatly increased risk of a THR into account, when confronted with the expiry of this period at some time between the ages of sixty and seventy, you will face, as shown in the previous paragraph, a demand for much higher premiums. This will most certainly be the case if, aged over sixty, you try to take out first-time cover, a strategy with relatively poor chances of a satisfactory outcome.

Even with steadily increasing premium rates, anyone interested in private medical insurance should start as young as possible, at a time in life when a good health record should qualify for relatively low premiums. Good insurers certainly reward loyalty over the long term; the promise to do so is one way of attracting young policy-holders, who, when it comes to insurance, are a low-risk category. This said, insurers still do their best to reserve their right to increase premiums every year, if the market and government regulations allow.

An insurer can also keep costs down by making special group arrangements with private hospitals, and this should be reflected in lower premiums. 'Own risk options' can also reduce premiums: a £100 'own risk' is often standard, and has the advantage of excluding small claims – always a high cost item for an insurer. The 'own risk' can, however, be as high as £2,000, in which case premiums should be very substantially reduced – but then you would be paying up to about a quarter of the costs of a THR. In every case it is a question of getting the sums right, as well as second-guessing future need for high-cost treatment (something the insurance companies tend to do better than their clients).

Unfortunately, although insurers are quick enough to exclude bad risks, they are not all that ready to reward good risks. If at the age of seventy, you have never had a day in bed for medical reasons, you will not gain that much benefit when taking out health cover. The most that can be said is that a good medical record will help keep exclusion clauses out of the policy, particularly when it comes to renewal. (Bear in mind that smokers are generally charged higher premiums.)

Some policies restrict cover to treatment where waiting time under the NHS exceeds a certain prescribed period, which may be anything from six to twelve weeks. This excludes cover for urgent cases, some of which may require intensive care, where patients receive priority treatment under the NHS. (Almost all accident and emergency treatment is excluded from private health cover, although long-term follow-up treatment may well be covered – just look at professional footballers.) Policies restricted to low-priority treatment carry a lower premium and are a particularly favourable form of cover for costly elective surgery such as THRs.

On the other hand, policies can include extra benefits such as covering the costs of convalescence, in exchange for higher premiums. All in all, there are any number of possible combinations, each with its own price tag. This means that for any condition requiring treatment, you are well advised first to consult your insurance company, if only to discover whether, and to what extent, costs are covered. (In relation to THRs, an insurance company is likely to have an upper limit, say £1,000, on the fee paid to the surgeon; anything above that figure you must then pay yourself.)

In any case, failure first to consult your insurance company may even affect your right to recover costs for which it would otherwise be liable. This is reasonable, since insurer companies have rules of procedure governing the choice of both specialists and hospitals; in both cases the company may only accept cases where a standard scale of charges has been agreed for the treatment required. In such cases the bills may be paid directly by the insurance company to hospitals and specialists who have agreed the standard terms. This category is almost certain to include such a standard operation as a THR. If you then choose a surgeon with fees above the agreed scale you will be charged separately for the amount of the excess.

11
Treatment Abroad

Every year about a million THRs are carried out world-wide. Of these, about 7 per cent – that is some 70,000 – will be in the United Kingdom, which has no more than 1 per cent of the world's population. Even so, in comparison with other EU countries, the number of THRs in the UK is low. In the Netherlands, with little more than a quarter of the population, the number is about a third that for the UK. At the same time, waiting lists in many parts of that country are as long as they are for NHS patients in the UK.

The Netherlands and the UK are probably exceptional within the EU for not being able to offer patients an appointment for a THR at short notice – say under a month. In both countries, however, waiting times vary considerably from one hospital to another. Patients waiting for a THR may be offered the alternative of treatment abroad, a process that has gone much further in the Netherlands than in the UK.

In contrast, hospitals in a number of EU countries, notably Germany, France, Belgium, Spain and Greece, are eager to welcome THR patients from outside their frontiers. These come mainly from other parts of the EU, particularly the Netherlands and the UK, with their long waiting lists.

For the five countries listed above with surplus capacity for THRs, this is the result not so much of government policy as of initiatives taken by specific hospitals. In other words, at least in certain regions in these countries, there are both orthopaedic surgeons looking for work and spare beds in the hospitals. To a degree this reflects over-investment in medical facilities: the teaching hospitals trained too many specialists in the 1980s and 1990s, and the number of hospital beds increased accordingly. This is not, however, comparable with private treatment in the UK. The rates charged by both the surgeons and the hospitals are not far above the level of the estimated costs of a THR on the NHS; occasionally they may even be lower.

In the UK, budget constraints make it certain that there is little surplus capacity in the NHS: it is no coincidence that the UK spends less than 7 per cent of GDP on health care, which is significantly lower than in other EU countries. (In Germany the figure is more than 10 per cent. In the Netherlands, government-imposed economies meant that from the 1980s onwards too few specialists were trained.) In 1980, when THRs were just beginning to come into their own, few foresaw the high level of demand that would arise from a steadily ageing population.

Implications of Having a THR Abroad

What does all this add up to for you as you wait for your THR? The probable answer is 'not very much'. The position may well change, however. So far the number of NHS patients receiving treatment abroad is less than 1 per cent, but to this must be added possible private patients.

The best publicized arrangement I am aware of is that made with a hospital in Lille, a large industrial town in the part of France closest to England. THR patients, who come from Kent, travel by train from Ashford International to Lille Europe in less than an hour. The hospital sees to it that they are looked after from the moment they arrive at the station in Lille.

Although essentially a French THR is the same as a British one, British patients will probably notice a number of differences, both medical and administrative, in hospital procedure. When it comes to the THR operation itself, the patient will probably be given a local rather than a general anaesthetic (see pages 91–5).

There may also be different procedures for reducing potential risks, such as deep vein thrombosis or bacterial infection. The latter could prove to be a considerable problem, since the stay in hospital could then be lengthened by several weeks. This is a serious matter, given that such infection occurs in about 3 per cent of all THRs.

This introduces one of the main problems you will face if you opt for treatment abroad. Although your every need is taken care of, this is not true of family and friends who want to visit and offer you comfort during your stay in hospital. Even from Ashford, going back and forth to Lille every day could be both tiring and expensive. Your husband, wife or children – or other potential visitors – would probably prefer to stay in a local hotel in Lille, but what can be done to pass the time outside hospital visiting hours? Lille is not really a tourist destination at any time of year.

If the NHS extends the scheme beyond Lille, other EU locations will be found with hospitals welcoming British THR patients, but none will be quite as convenient for patients from Kent. For one thing, most other locations will involve returning by air to the UK after the operation, which is not as simple as travelling by Eurostar.

Private Treatment Abroad

If NHS patients are limited to specific arrangements made with hospitals in other parts of the EU, with private treatment you have a free choice, not necessarily confined to the EU. Given the relatively high price of such treatment within the UK, this may well be the way to lower costs. The problem is the sheer diversity of what is on offer.

Every EU country has its own mainstream system of health care, governed by its complex of bureaucratic regulation. Since, however, private treatment falls outside such systems, price structures, even within a single country, have no fixed form. If as a British patient the cost of private treatment locally is of the order of

£8,000, you may do considerably better in some other EU country. At this price level, however, you would be well advised first to exhaust the possibilities of treatment within the UK.

Once the cost of travel, including that of supporting family or friends, is taken into account, the hidden costs of a THR abroad are likely to make it a poor buy. It will only be a viable alternative where there is some particular factor that makes it advantageous for you as an individual. This could be close family residing in a given foreign location, for example; a British widow or widower looking for a THR might well choose an EU country in which a grown-up child was working.

The European Court

In July 2001, the European Court reached a decision that has far-reaching implications that have yet to be worked out. Although it did not directly relate to THR, it could well change the position of THR patients, particularly under the NHS, when it comes to seeking treatment outside the UK.

The European Court decided in favour of two Dutch residents, who, unknown to each other, had gone outside the Netherlands for medical treatment, which they claimed the Dutch Insurance Funds should pay for. Although neither case related to arthritis of the hip, the principle on which the cases were decided could relate to cases of residents of one EU country having a THR in another. For UK residents, the question to be answered is simple: is the judgement of the European Court sufficiently wide in its scope to allow a British patient to claim repayment from the NHS of the costs of a THR carried in an EU hospital outside the United Kingdom?

Quite apart from the legal principles involved, one significant fact is worth noting. Not only were the two Dutch claimants and the insurance funds to which they belonged represented before the Court, but twelve governments of EU countries also exercised their right, under EU law, to present their views. Only Greece and Spain chose not to be represented: the UK, on the other hand briefed not one but two lawyers to argue its case.

The only explanation is that the legal advice given to the NHS was that the case, if decided in favour of the two Dutch claimants, would radically affect the rights of British patients to medical treatment abroad at the cost of the NHS. This could go as far as allowing an NHS patient to reclaim the costs of a THR carried out in any part of the EU. As of writing, the NHS may allow such a claim only if you have been waiting for longer than a year for your operation.

If the Dutch case had related to a THR, the claim for repayment of costs could well have failed, for the simple reason that 'satisfactory and adequate treatment was available in the Netherlands at an establishment having contractual arrangements with the sickness insurance fund'. If the claim had been that of a UK resident, the NHS would almost certainly have based its case on a similar principle. However, in a case now going through the courts, the claimant is arguing that treatment available only after waiting for a period of several months is neither satisfactory nor adequate.

The refusal on the part of the NHS to pay the costs of a THR performed outside the UK depends on legislation at national level. It is, however, a fundamental principle of the EU that its own law takes precedence over that of any member state. (The European Court has overruled a number of decisions of the House of Lords, for example.)

Health Care Bureaucracy

When it comes to the administration of public health care, every EU member state has its own system, supported by a vast bureaucracy (of which that of the British NHS is the largest). Although in the UK politicians and the media are accustomed to bashing the NHS, at the same time praising the presumed advantages of alternative systems in other parts of the EU, when it comes to basics all these systems, including the NHS, suffer from the same problems.

One thing they all have in common is to consolidate the financial issues at the level of a generalized condition treated by institutions operating on a large scale. This means, for example, standardized charges that do not take into account variations between individual cases; on the financial side it makes no difference to the NHS whether a THR takes one hour or four, although this may upset a hospital timetable. All that an NHS hospital needs to know is the number of THRs that its budget allows for in its accounting year.

In the 2001 case, the Dutch Insurance Funds made it clear that they worked with a system of 'benefits in kind under which an insured person is entitled not to reimbursement of costs incurred for medical treatment but to free treatment'. Essentially this is the position under the NHS. As far as the patient is concerned, no money changes hands: all the accounting goes on behind the scenes, on the basis of vast global sums sluicing back and forth within the medical bureaucracy.

The NHS, in rejecting a claim for repayment of the costs of a THR performed outside the UK, would be little concerned about the actual money involved (which could well not involve it in any loss at all), but about the time that its officials would have to spend in dealing with each individual case. The deviant or isolated case is anathema to any bureaucracy.

This leads to another argument against recognizing such cases, which can be called opening the floodgates. The NHS could well concede that the odd special case would not cause it all that much trouble: any sound system of administration must have a certain amount of flexibility. The problem with a rule such as that established by the European Court in July 2001 is that it leaves the way open to any number of claims – no one can tell how many. If half the British patients waiting for a THR were to make their own arrangements with hospitals outside the UK, and then after the operation present the bill to the NHS, a whole new department might have to be opened to deal with the claims for repayment. Perish the thought!

This was clearly in the minds of the Dutch Insurance

Funds when they chose to contest the cases of the two patients claiming repayment of the costs of treatment outside the Netherlands. Adapting the words recorded in the judgment of the European Court to a possible British claim, then:

> if insured persons were at liberty, regardless of the circumstances, to use the services of hospitals outside the NHS, whether they were situated in the United Kingdom or in another Member State, all the planning which goes into the NHS in an effort to guarantee a rationalized, stable, balanced and accessible supply of hospital services would be jeopardized at a stroke.

One can almost hear the Secretary of State uttering the words cited above in answer to a parliamentary question, though the description of the supply of hospital services by the NHS as 'rationalized, stable, balanced and accessible' might well provoke hoots of laughter from the opposition benches . . .

EU Law and THRs

So much for the administrative aspects of the case at hand: what then, does the law have to say?

Applying these the two relevant Articles of the European Community Treaty in the context of this book, orthopaedic surgeons performing THRs in the EU but outside the UK may not be subject to any restrictions on their freedom to operate on a UK resident. The question then, is, would the refusal of the NHS to pay the costs of such an operation amount to a restriction on the freedom of EU surgeons established outside the UK to practise their profession? This, after all, is what the two Dutch Insurance Funds did when insured patients claimed the costs of medical treatment outside the Netherlands.

The question, ultimately, is one of medical necessity. Whatever these words mean, they certainly describe any genuine case of a patient waiting for a THR. Then, adapting the words of the final judgment of the Court to the position of a British patient, the NHS could only refuse to authorize treatment abroad, 'if the same or equally effective treatment can be obtained without undue delay' within the NHS.

The British government, in the course of 2002, acknowledged that delays of more than six months were not acceptable. If, then, the waiting time for a THR is longer than six months (which at the time of writing is the general case under the NHS), effective treatment cannot be obtained 'without due delay'. Patients, therefore, who find treatment abroad 'without undue delay' can send the bill to the NHS. The only problem is that the NHS claims that 'undue delay' means longer than a year.

If you are waiting for a THR in the UK, I would be very wary about advising you to try the strategy of being operated on in some other EU member state, in the hope of the costs being paid by the NHS. When, in 2001, I tried to adopt the same strategy within the Dutch health insurance system, I met considerable resistance. My insurers would have accepted a group arrangement agreed, on their initiative, with a British hospital; what they could not accept was an individual patient making his own arrangements for a THR operation in the UK. Even though this was precisely what happened in the two cases decided by the European Court in July 2001, my insurance company showed no sign of accepting the implications of this decision. As the case now going through the courts demonstrates, if you, as a UK resident, were to try the same strategy as I did, you would almost certainly encounter resistance on the same scale on the part of the NHS.

Plainly, for the great majority of patients waiting for a THR under the NHS, all this is asking too much. The odd patient, however, will have contacts in other EU states, and in an easily accessible country such as Belgium, it is surprisingly simple to make a provisional appointment for a THR to be carried out within a month or two. Even so, the NHS bureaucracy, confronted with this possibility – and knowing that it is already paying for THRs in Lille – still refuses to concede individual cases. It may not be able to do so much longer. In a case brought by a THR patient, and heard in the High Court on 1 October 2003, it was ruled that patients facing 'undue delay' because of long NHS waiting lists were entitled under European law to obtain funding for overseas treatment. The case may well end up in the House of Lords, but even so I predict that the High Court judgment will stand.

Alternatively, with the much wider choice of hospitals promised by the British government in 2002, patients could well be offered THRs, within reasonable time, in

NHS hospitals outside their own region. It is then up to the individual patient to decide whether this is acceptable.

All in all, operations in other EU states are unlikely to become an important part of the THR scene. They are at best a stop-gap measure, at least if the British government's promised improvements to the NHS are actually realized.

THR for British Residents Abroad

There is one final point. The position dealt with in this chapter could be reversed. If, after long residence in the UK, you choose to live abroad in another EU state – preferring, say, the climate of Provence to that of the Cotswolds – you are very likely to forfeit your right to treatment under the NHS in the UK (even though you paid the premiums for years).

Urgent treatment, while abroad, is covered by mutual arrangements within the EU, provided that you as an NHS patient follow the correct bureaucratic procedures. This is fine if you have an accident or fall ill while on holiday, but it will not help with a THR.

Provence could well be fine as a place to live, but you may still refer the good old NHS when it comes to major surgery, such as a THR. Forget it. In practice you can only come back to the UK for elective surgery as a private patient. You know what this involves from reading Chapter 10. In any case, why worry? Except possibly for the Netherlands, no other EU state has the sort of waiting lists for a THR that you find as an NHS patient. One small blessing as a result of moving abroad is that you do not have to wait long for a THR in your local hospital. You may even find that many of the doctors and nurses can speak English, and the food will almost certainly be better!

12
The Future of THR

Considering the present state of the art in THRs, there seems to be little room for improvement. As long ago as 1983, Henry Mankin, in his presidential address to the American Orthopedic Association, stated that 'mechanical engineering is near the end of its possible improvements and additions to our caretaking systems'. Writing at the turn of the new millennium, he had not changed his views, noting, however, that 'the engineers continue to provide us with new devices and new approaches to our problems'.

It is now accepted that the basic design of the prosthesis, described in Chapter 5, leaves little room for improvement. Nevertheless, no year goes by without modifications being introduced by medical suppliers, often supported by articles in medical journals explaining the advantages claimed for them. While some orthopaedic surgeons have little doubt about which models are best (even to the point of having their patients pay much higher prices), others accept that there is little to choose between the models offered by the market. According to one orthopaedic surgeon, 'the justification for so many designs is elusive, perhaps representing commercial or egotistical interests rather than a desire for improvement in patient care'.

One problem is that the thirty years that have elapsed since the basic Charnley prosthesis came to be generally accepted have hardly been sufficient for conclusive follow-up studies. The wide variety of prostheses available, together with continual small changes in operative techniques, make the value of such studies even more problematic.

Even if one particular prosthesis were better than the alternatives, its use could be so restricted that the statistical results justifying the claims made for it could still fail to meet strict scientific standards. It is just like trying to decide what is the best car, or the best airline: too many factors, many of them changing almost every year, must be taken into account to justify any one conclusion.

In October 2003, a number of British consultants announced through the media a radical change in the surgery of THR. The new keyhole approach would require two small incisions, of which the longest would only be 4 cm. The much reduced level of operative trauma then makes for a much more rapid recovery, with the patient leaving hospital only a day after the operation. Many surgeons are sceptical, simply because it takes five years to tell whether a new untried procedure is effective. The key factor is the length of time a patient can live with an implant before revision surgery is necessary. With conventional surgery this period can be twenty years or even more: if, with the new procedure, this period proves to be substantially shorter, few surgeons will be likely to adopt it.

Quite radical improvements may come from the newly developing world of 'tissue engineering'. THR takes for granted the non-reactive, inorganic prosthesis, made of metal, plastics and ceramics. The limitations of any such prosthesis are inherent in the materials out of which it is made. The alternative, so far unrealized in the field of THR, is to work with an organic implant, in its original form quite different in structure to the bone tissue to be replaced, but so designed as to become identical to the parent tissue. Inherent in this process are all the familiar problems of organ transplants, including rejection by the patient's immune system.

One way of dealing with this is to use a patient's own tissue, a technique used in other types of orthopaedic surgery – particularly the treatment of some forms of trauma. At the same time, it is significant that THR patients are commonly asked to donate the bone tissue removed from their hips (although this may be required for purposes unrelated to THRs). Even so, current research includes the search for safe immunosuppressive agents that would make it possible for a patient to accept bone tissue from a donor. Success here would greatly increase the possibility of a THR based on human bone tissue being accepted by the patient as if it were from his own body.

Fundamental to progress of this kind is the fact that:

the original concept of external tissue/organ culture, followed by surgical implantation, is already being modified in favour of a method whereby biomaterials, with the correct geometry, are implanted in the recipient site to be colonized by the local cells. This route for tissue regeneration circumvents many of the problems of the external culture method and may lead to a completely new form of restorative orthopaedic surgery this century where plastics and alloys of metals will have little place.

These words, published in 2001 by Neil Rushton, a British orthopaedic surgeon, probably state the ultimate position envisaged by current research. Whether the future of THR suggested by them would be a real improvement in the well-being of actual patients is another matter altogether.

In a quite different direction, continued research might lead to medicines effective in slowing down or even stopping degeneration as a result of arthritic disease. Medicinal treatment is already used for rheumatoid arthritis and localized cartilage defects, but these conditions account for only a very small number of THRs.

Bibliography

V.H. Frankel and M. Nordin, *Basic Biomechanics of the Skeletal System*, Lea & Fabiger, 1980.

A. Gawande, 'When doctors make mistakes', *New Yorker*, 1 February 1999, pp. 40–55 [5].

V. Grove, 'I need new mountains to climb', *The Times*, 16 April 2002.

P. Hutton and G. Cooper, 'Fundamental Principles and Practice of Anaesthesia', *The Evolution of Orthopaedic Surgery* (ed. L. Kleneman), Royal Society of Medicine Press, 2001.

Kans patient op infectie in ziekenhuis, *NRC Handelsblad*, 13 Augustus 2001.

R. Klapper & L. Huey, *Heal Your Hips: How to Prevent Hip Surgery – and What to Do If You Need It*, Wiley, 1999.

L. Kleneman, 'Arthroplasty of the hip', *The Evolution of Orthopaedic Surgery*, pp. 1–12.

L. Kleneman, 'Setting the scene – the start of

orthopaedic surgery', *The Evolution of Orthopaedic Surgery*, pp. 1–12.

H.J. Mankin, 'Orthopaedics in 2050: a look at the future', *The Evolution of Orthopaedic Surgery*, pp. 1–12.

D.A. Miller, 'Orthopaedic product technology during the second half of the twentieth century', *The Evolution of Orthopaedic Surgery*, pp. 221–8.

Jim Northcott, *Britain's Future*, Policy Studies Institute, London, 1999.

S.B. Nuland, 'When doctors get it wrong', *New York Review of Books,* 18 July 2002, pp. 10–13 [5].

J. O'Connor, 'Biomechanics', in *The Evolution of Orthopaedic Surgery*, pp. 1–12.

T. Stuttaford, 'Risks overcome in rapid recovery', *The Times*, 12 January 2002 [5].

R. Villar, *Hip Replacement: A Patient's Guide to Surgery and Recovery*, Granta, 1995.

W. Waugh, *John Charnley: The Man and the Hip*, London, Springer-Verlag, 1990.

References

Introduction: the quotation at the head of the chapter comes from D.A. Miller, 'Orthopaedic product technology during the second half of the twentieth century', in *The Evolution of Orthopaedic Surgery* (ed. L. Kleneman, Royal Society of Medicine Press, 2001), pp. 221–8.

Chapter 1: Figures 1 and 2 come from V.H. Frankel and M. Nordin, *Basic Biomechanics of the Skeletal System*, Lea & Fabiger, 1980, p. 156, 157. The quotations ['lightly loaded . . .] on page 17 come from pages 77, 78 of the same book. The report (page 24) on *rituximab* comes from *The Times*, 26 October 2002.

Chapter 2: The report on Celebrex (page 30) comes from NRC Handelsblad, 20 July 2002, Wetenschap en Onderwijs, p. 6.

In London go to the Yoga Therapy Centre, 90 Pentonville Road, N1 9HS. Tel. 020 7689 3040.

Chapter 3: The words quoted on page 42 ['doomed to

failure . . .] come from W. Waugh, *John Charnley: The Man and the Hip*, London, Springer-Verlag, 1990, p. 100, those quoted on page 44 ['inherently slippery . . .'] from p. 105, on page 47 ['old age . . .'] from p. 108, on page 47 ['mobility and stability are incompatible . . .'] on p. 111, on and page 51 ['deceptively easy to perform . . .'] from p. 226.

Charnley's two papers, cited on page 49, are to be found in *Clinical Orthopaedics* 1970:72:7–21 and *Journal of Bone and Joint Surgery* (British) 1972:54:61–76. The editorial quoted on page 52 is to be found in the *British Medical Journal* 1987:195:514.

Chapter 5: The Birmingham Hip Replacement has its own website, www.midmedtech.co.uk (which provided much of the material for this section). For Finsbury Orthopaedics see www.finsbury.org.

Chapter 6: The figures for the number of THRs performed by orthopaedic surgeons were provided by the Health Services Management Centre, Birmingham University, as reported in *The Times*, 25 May 2002.

Chapter 7: The words quoted ['inherent uncertainty . . .'] on page 68 come from the *New York Review of Books*, 18 July 2002, p. 10. Those ['actual negligence . . .'] on page 76 come from A. Gawande, 'When doctors make mistakes', *New Yorker*, 1 February 1999, pp. 40–55, p. 44.

The figures cited on page 69, which come from the Government Actuary's Department, have probably improved in the last five years.

Starting with the first volume in 1990 professional witnesses, mostly consultants, are all listed in the cases

References 181

to be found in the *Medical Law Reports* (see page 77).

Chapter 8: The report (page 133) about Gillian Lynne's will-power comes from *The Times*, 16 April 2002.

Chapter 9: The figures relating to the decline in the number of elderly patients in NHS hospitals, and the increase in the number in private health care institutions, come from Jim Northcott, *Britain's Future*, Policy Studies Institute, London 1999.

Chapter 10: The report on page 140 ['first call on a consultant's time . . .'] comes from *The Daily Telegraph*, 13 June 2002 p. 2. The sum of £4,000 for an NHS hip replacement (page 141) is reported in *The Times*, 16 April 2002, p. 12. The 'Good Hospital Guide' published as a supplement to the *Sunday Times* (6 April 2003) lists the cost of THRs in some 150 private hospitals. For further information see also www.nuffieldhospitals.org.uk or www.bupa.co.uk and the guides published by the Association of British Insurers entitled, 'Are you buying private medical insurance?' The 150,000 operations a year to be contracted out to private hospitals (page 149) are reported in the *Independent*, 19 April 2002, p. 6. The figures for tax and NI contributions (page 151) are reported in the *Independent*, 18 April 2002, p. 20.

Chapter 11: The words quoted ['sickness insurance fund . . .'] on page 164 comes from the official report of the Judgment of the European Court, 12 July 2001 (1), p. 6, those on page 166 ['to free treatment . . .'] from page 2, those on page 167 ['jeopardized at a stroke . . .'] from page 11, those on page 168 ['without undue delay . . .'] from page 15.

The relevant EU community law is based on what are

now Articles 49 and 50 of the European Community Treaty, as amended in Amsterdam in 1998.

Article 49 provides, quite simply, that 'restrictions on freedom to provide services within the Community shall be prohibited in respect of nationals of Member States who are established in a State of the Community other than that of the person for whom the services are intended'.

By Article 50, 'Services shall be considered to be "services" . . . where they are normally provided for remuneration . . . [and] in particular include activities of the professions'.

Chapter 12: the words quoted on page 172 ['caretaking systems . . .'] and on page 174 ['tissue engineering . . .'] come from H.J. Mankin, 'Orthopaedics in 2050: a look at the future', in *The Evolution of Orthopaedic Surgery* (ed. L. Kleneman, Royal Society of Medicine Press, 2001), pp. 1–12. Those quoted on page 173 ['patient care . . .'] and on page 175 ['metals will have little place'] come from the chapter by Rushton in *The Evolution of Orthopaedic Surgery* (ed. L. Kleneman, Royal Society of Medicine Press, 2001, pp. 83, 88).

Index

Figures in italics refer to illustrations